HEALTHCARE SIMULATION

HEALTHCARE SIMULATION

A Guide for Operations Specialists

Edited by

LAURA T. GANTT
East Carolina University College of Nursing, Greenville, NC, USA

H. MICHAEL YOUNG
Level 3 Healthcare, Mesa, AZ, USA

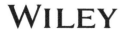

For general information on our other products and services or for technical support, please contact our
Customer Care Department within the United States at (800) 762-2974, outside the United States at
(317) 572-3993 or fax (317) 572-4002.

Wiley also publishes its books in a variety of electronic formats. Some content that appears in print may
not be available in electronic formats. For more information about Wiley products, visit our web site at
www.wiley.com.

Library of Congress Cataloging-in-Publication Data:

Healthcare simulation : a guide for operations specialists / edited by Laura T. Gantt, H. Michael Young.
    p. ; cm.
  Includes bibliographical references and index.
  ISBN 978-1-118-94941-2 (hardback)
I. Gantt, Laura, 1957–, editor.   II. Young, H. Michael, 1960–, editor.
[DNLM: 1. Education, Medical.   2. Clinical Competence.   3. Educational Technology.
4. Health Personnel–education.   5. Patient Simulation. W 18]
  R834
  610.71–dc23

                                                                                2015036801

Set in 10/12pt Times by SPi Global, Pondicherry, India

10 9 8 7 6 5 4 3 2 1

1 2016

This book is dedicated to the memory of Joshua C. Brehm.

Laura T. Gantt

For her patience, support, and enduring love, I dedicate this book to my wonderful wife, Nora L. Young. Thank you for the past 30 years, and the life that awaits us. I can't imagine it without you.

H. Michael Young

CONTENTS

CONTRIBUTORS LIST

Guillaume Alinier, PhD, MPhys, PGCert, CPhys, MIPEM, MInstP, SFHEA, NTF University of Hertfordshire, Hatfield, UK

S. Scott Atkinson, BBA, NREMT-P Summa Health, Akron, OH, USA

Evan J. Bartley, BS ECU College of Nursing, Greenville, NC, USA

Timothy R. Brock, PhD, CPT, ID(S&L+) The Institute 4 Worthy Performance LLC, Winter Park, FL, USA; The ROI Institute, Birmingham, AL, USA; The Institute for Performance Improvement L3C, Chicago, IL, USA; Full Sail University, Winter Park, FL, USA; Webster University, St Louis, MO, USA; and Franklin University, Columbus, OH USA

Adam Dodson, NRP, CCEMT-P, NCEE Johns Hopkins Medicine Simulation Center, Baltimore, MD, USA

Thomas A. Dongilli, AT, CHSOS Winter Institute for Simulation Education and Research (WISER), Pittsburgh, PA, USA

Laura T. Gantt, PhD, RN, CEN, NE-BC East Carolina University College of Nursing, Greenville, NC, USA

Jesika S. Gavilanes, MA Oregon Health & Science University, Portland, OR, USA

Gene W. Hobbs University of North Carolina, Chapel Hill, NC, USA

Mary Holtschneider, RN-BC, BSN, MPA, NREMT-P, CPLP Durham VA Medical Center, Durham, NC, USA

Cheryl Hunter, BSN, RN Tarleton State University, Stephensville, TX, USA

Valeriy Kozmenko, MD Parry Center for Clinical Skills and Simulation, Sioux Falls, SD, USA

Amar Patel, DHSc, MS, NRP WakeMed Health & Hospitals, Raleigh, NC, USA

Morgan Scherwitz, MSN, RN Hendrick Medical Center, Abilene, TX, USA

Lindsey Scott, MSN, RN Consultant, Austin, TX, USA

Emily Shaw, MA, CMI, EMT-B Mimic Technologies, Simugreat, SAGES, Baltimore, MD, USA

H. Michael Young, BBS, MDiv, CHSE Level 3 Healthcare, Mesa, AZ, USA

CONTRIBUTORS BIOS

Guillaume Alinier, PhD, MPhys, PGCert, CPhys, MIPEM, MInstP, SFHEA, NTF, has worked in the field of healthcare simulation education, research, and facility design for the last 15 years. He obtained a Master in Applied Physics from the University of Portsmouth (UK) and his PhD from the University of Hertfordshire (UK). He holds a full professorship from Hertfordshire where he setup and directed a large simulation center designed for undergraduate and postgraduate interprofessional activities. He holds a visiting position with Northumbria University in Newcastle, UK, since 2009. His primary position at present is with Hamad Medical Corporation Ambulance Service (Doha, Qatar) as Assistant Executive Director of Research; he also helped revamp the training program of paramedics. Since the start of his career in healthcare simulation, Dr. Alinier has received several awards from the UK Higher Education Academy (NTF 2006, SFHEA 2009) for his work in teaching and learning with students, for mentoring colleagues, and supporting the development of several simulation centers around the world. He is a regular keynote speaker at international conferences and has published extensively. He has been chair or co-chair of major simulation conferences, such as ASPiH 2007, SESAM 2008, and IMSH 2012. He is actively involved with the simulation societies through various roles, including the International Nursing Association for Clinical Simulation in Nursing (INACSL) as a member of its Standards Advisory Board and the Society for Simulation in Healthcare (SSH) as member of the CHSOS Certification Committee, Program Accreditation Council, and Meetings Oversight Committee.

S. Scott Atkinson, BBA, NREMT-P, began his career as a basic EMT and firefighter, while moving forward with his EMT advanced and paramedic certifications. He has worked in the field as a paramedic in the inner-city and as part of the Critical Care

Transport Team in many areas of Ohio, West Virginia and Pennsylvania. He is certified as a Basic Life Support (BLS) and Advanced Cardiac Life Support (ACLS) instructor, and has also served as a Tech Level III Hazmat Team Member and 240 hr firefighter. He started, and still actively manages and runs, the Virtual Care Simulation Labs at Summa Health System and is currently building a new simulation center through a 1.5 million dollar state grant. He holds an Associate's Degree in Information Technology and is currently working toward the completion of his Bachelor's degree in Business Administration. Mr. Atkinson belongs to many simulation user groups and was past chair of the Society for Simulation in Healthcare's (SSH) Simulation Operations and Technology Section (SOTS). Mr. Atkinson is a prominent simulation technologist and educator and has been instrumental in several educational development programs, as well as new simulation center start-ups. He has developed and is preparing for the start of the first simulation technologists' associate degree program through the University of Akron to begin in the spring of 2016. He will teach from a specially designed simulation lab that he and his team had designed and built for simulation technology instruction. Mr. Atkinson is an entrepreneur and has designed and built a cardiac simulator with his simulation team, which was recently licensed through a prominent simulation company. In his free time, he is a real estate agent and also owns and operates several businesses.

Evan J. Bartley, BS, has worked in the field of instructional technology over the last 5 years at East Carolina University (ECU) College of Nursing. He began working as a simulation technologist and has stepped into a managerial role, supervising not only the support of simulation technologies, but distance education and other instructional technologies. Mr. Bartley received a Bachelor's degree from ECU in 2009 in Information and Computer Technology with a concentration in Information Security. Mr. Bartley is currently working on his Master's at ECU in Instructional Technology and is COMPTIA Security+ certified.

Timothy R. Brock, PhD, CPT, ID(S&L+), is the CEO of the Institute 4 Worthy Performance, a Practice Leader with the Institute for Performance Improvement (TIfPI), and an Associate with the ROI Institute. He is a Certified Performance Technologist (CPT) with the International Society for Performance Improvement (ISPI) and a Certified Instructional Designer with a specialization in Simulation and Labs (ID(S&L+)) with TIfPI. Dr. Brock earned his PhD at Capella University in Education with a specialization in training and performance improvement. He is a retired air force field grade officer who began using advanced simulation technologies for training and education in 1979. He retired from Lockheed Martin Global Training and Logistics in 2012 where he was the manager of their Science of Learning and Performance Improvement team for global military and healthcare learning and simulation training solutions. He is a member of the Society for Simulation in Healthcare and serves on two committees: the Technology and Standards Committee and the Preparatory Materials Committee for the Healthcare Simulation Operations Specialist certification. Dr. Brock is also a member of the CPT Oversight Sub-Committee with ISPI. He is a published author and frequent international conference speaker. He can be reached at Tim@ti4wp.com.

Adam Dodson, NRP, CCEMT-P, NCEE, has been in Emergency Medicine and Emergency Medical Services (EMS) for over 20 years. He obtained his Paramedic Degree and License through Cecil College and began teaching in 1997 for the U.S. Army Medical Department Center and School (AMEDDC&S). Adam's career with Johns Hopkins Hospital began in 1997 as a Critical Care Paramedic. He was instrumental in the development of new employees as a field training officer. He started using simulation and teaching in 2003 with the University of Maryland and University of Maryland—Baltimore County (UMBC). Adam has taught interdisciplinary hospital team members for more than a decade and is the Lead Simulation Specialist at the Johns Hopkins Medicine Simulation Center. He often meets with clients from foreign countries and discusses challenges of teaching in austere environments or creating simulation centers. He has worked on international projects with the Johns Hopkins Program for International Education in Gynecology and Obstetrics (JHPIEGO), the United States Agency for International Development (USAID), the United States Department of Defense, Johns Hopkins International (JHI), and Johns Hopkins International Global Services. In 2015, he assisted in the launch of a train-the-trainer program in Nigeria. Adam serves as a technical advisor for the Johns Hopkins University Biomedical Department, creating several low-cost task trainers for countries around the globe. Adam also chairs the Benchmarking Subcommittee for Hospital-Based Section of the Society for Simulation in Healthcare (SSH), and he is the Vice-Chair of the Simulation Operations and Technology Section. He has spoken at several conferences on innovations in simulation and pushing the boundaries of technology.

Thomas A. Dongilli, AT, CHSOS, has worked in the healthcare simulation industry for over 21 years. Tom is the Director of Operations at the Peter M. Winter Institute for Simulation, Education and Research (WISER). In this role, Tom supplies operational leadership to WISER's main facility and its' seven satellite centers: WISER has been providing simulation services since 1994. Prior to this role, Tom was the Chief Anesthesia Technologist for the University of Pittsburgh Medical Center. Tom has extensive experience in simulation center design, integration, and operations and has designed simulation centers both nationally and internationally. He also contributes expert knowledge and experience in the practical design, implementation, operation, and monitoring of simulation based facilities and medical learning systems. Some of Tom's published works include chapters in *A Manual of Simulation in Healthcare* and *Concepts, Trends, and Possibilities for Using Clinical Simulation in Nursing Education*. Tom has also authored many courses pertaining to simulation center operations, including TechSim, Designing Your Simulation Center, and Operational Best Practices for Your Simulation Center. Tom's area of clinical interest is in the field of *in situ* simulations and patient safety; he has created simulation-based programs for Mock Codes, Clinical Site Assessments and most recently authored a course called "The First 5 minutes, What to do Until the Code Team Arrives." Tom was the 2014 International Meeting for Simulation in Healthcare planning committee co-chair. Tom has been an active member of the Society for Simulation in Healthcare since its inception. Tom currently has a role in the following committees with the Society for Simulation in Healthcare: CHSOS Exam Prep committee and the Oversight Committee. Tom was the lead author on the creation of the Society for Simulation in Healthcare's Policy and Procedure manual.

Laura T. Gantt, PhD, RN, CEN, NE-BC, is an Associate Professor and Interim Associate Dean for Nursing Support Services in the College of Nursing. She began her formal work with healthcare simulation in 2006 when she was hired to establish simulation and teaching labs in the new East Carolina College of Nursing building. The departments under her supervision include the Concepts Integration Labs, Learning Resource Center, Instructional Technology, Student Development and Counseling, and Student Services. Laura has published a number of journal articles and book chapters on simulation and emergency nursing topics. She developed the outline for this book and then began searching for a technology expert to co-author it. She and Michael Young met in March of 2013. She has served on the CHSOS Committee since April of 2013. Previous to the time that she went to work at ECU, Laura was an administrator for the emergency, ambulatory, and transport service line at Pitt Country Memorial Hospital (now Vidant Medical Center); she still practices as a staff nurse in Vidant's Minor Emergency Department. Laura is a Certified Emergency Nurse (CEN) and also holds a certification as a nurse executive (NE-BC). She has a BSN from Duke University, MSN from the University of North Carolina, and a PhD in Nursing from the University of Colorado.

Jesika S. Gavilanes, MA, is currently the OHSU Simulation Operations Director for the Oregon Health & Science University Simulation Center in the Collaborative Life Sciences Building (CLSB). She has worked at the Oregon Health & Science University (OHSU) for over 18 years. She has been involved with simulation operations since 2002. She first became a simulation technician in 2003 and now oversees a team of seven simulation operation specialists. She completed her Masters in Teaching at Portland State University in August of 2008. In her role as Operations Director, Ms. Gavilanes oversees the operations of the 20,000 sq. ft. Interprofessional OHSU Simulation Center. She is the current Chair of the Oregon Simulation Alliance and has led the efforts of developing and implementing a Statewide Sim Tech Academy, educating over 80 sim techs across the state and Pacific Northwest. Ms. Gavilanes has been involved with simulation facilities across the country assisting with logistics, operations, and simulation implementation for the past 10 years. She currently is serving her third year as the Chair for the Society for Simulation in Healthcare Technical Operations Track. Ms. Gavilanes is also a member of the International Nursing Association for Clinical Simulation and Learning (INACSL).

Gene W. Hobbs has worked within the healthcare simulation field for 13 years, first at Duke University Medical Center, and then at the University of North Carolina at Chapel Hill (UNC-CH). In his faculty role at UNC, Gene serves as a clinical instructor for the Department of Pediatrics and Associate Director of Simulation for the School of Medicine focusing on interprofessional education throughout campus. Research has been an integral part of Gene's career that started as a research technician and Certified Hyperbaric Technologist 22 years ago. Gene is a Founding Board Member of the Rubicon Foundation, Inc.; he is also project manager for their Research Repository, which earned him the 2010 DAN/Rolex Diver of the Year Award. Gene has authored or co-authored 14 peer reviewed articles and over 50 abstracts. Gene's most recent publication in Critical Care Medicine with Dr. Noa Segall and colleagues utilized simulation to evaluate patient load effects on response time to critical arrhythmias in cardiac telemetry.

Mary Holtschneider, RN-BC, BSN, MPA, NREMT-P, CPLP, is Simulation Education Coordinator at the U.S. Department of Veterans Affairs, Durham VA Medical Center in Durham, North Carolina. She also serves as the Veterans Integrated Service Network (VISN) 6 Simulation Champion and Co-Director of the Durham VA Inteprofessional Advanced Fellowship in Clinical Simulation. She frequently writes and speaks on simulation-related topics and is the Simulation Columnist for the Journal for Nurses in Professional Development. Her areas of simulation interest include hospital *in situ* training, interprofessional team communication and team development, stroke/cardiac emergency response, and using simulation for process and quality improvement initiatives.

Cheryl Hunter, BSN, RN, received her BSN from Tarleton State University (TSU) in 2008 and began her nursing career in emergency nursing, where she continued to practice until 2013. Ms. Hunter accepted her current position as the Simulation Lab Supervisor at TSU, Department of Nursing in 2012. Ms. Hunter has been one of the leads in the development of the new Center for Clinical Simulation and Competency (CCSC). She has participated in a number of simulation-focused research projects and has presented at the International Meeting for Simulation in Healthcare (SSH) as a member of a discussion panel and poster presenter. Ms. Hunter is currently working toward her MSN. Most recently, Cheryl received the Tarleton State University Enhancing the Student Experience Award for her work in developing and implementing a multi-agency, community-based mass casualty disaster simulation.

Valeriy Kozmenko, MD, graduated from Lugansk State Medical University (Ukraine) in 1992 and obtained training in Anesthesiology and Critical Care. After moving to the United States, Dr. Kozmenko worked at Louisiana State University Health Sciences Center since 2002 and was soon promoted as Director of Human Patient Simulation. His scholarly activities include more than 50 presentations and publications and seven book chapters; his scholarly activities have been well recognized in the international simulation community. In 2013, Dr. Kozmenko was awarded a patent on an innovative medical simulation computer system that he developed. Since October of 2013, Dr. Kozmenko has served as the Director of the Parry Center for Clinical Skills and Simulation at the University of South Dakota Sanford School of Medicine. In 2015, the Society for Simulation in Healthcare recognized Dr. Kozmenko and Brian Wallenburg with the fifth place award for developing and implementing an innovative simulation scenario programming concept.

Amar Patel, DHSc, MS, NRP, is the director for the Center for Innovative Learning at WakeMed Health & Hospitals in Raleigh, North Carolina. He is a nationally registered paramedic and received his BA from Goucher College, an MS from UMBC, and his DHSc from Nova Southeastern University. Prior to becoming the director for the Center for Innovative Learning in 2007, Dr. Patel served as an advanced life support program instructor and the project manager of medical simulation for the Maryland Fire and Rescue Institute at the University of Maryland, College Park. In this role he was responsible for developing new curriculum, as well as integrating simulation methodology and the technology into all of the advanced life support (ALS) programs. He was the lead developer of simulation scenarios and the technical simulation expert at the local and state level. Today, Dr. Patel is an editorial board member for Carolina Fire Rescue EMS Journal. He has published many articles on simulation center architectural design, program administration, and audiovisual design. He continues to provide consultation for programs looking to integrate the simulation methodology or expand the utilization of simulation technology. Dr. Patel is involved in simulation-based research that focuses on integration and implementation of simulation as means to improve human and system processes. Dr. Patel was a contributing author for *Defining Excellence in Simulation Programs*, published by Wolters Klumer in 2014.

Morgan Scherwitz, MSN, RN, is the Nurse Manager of the Antenatal Triage Unit at Hendrick Hospital in Abilene, TX. She received her BSN from York College of Pennsylvania and her MSN from Liberty University before becoming Laboratory Manager at Tarleton State University in Stephenville, TX. After 6 years of creating and overseeing the simulation and nursing skills labs at Tarleton State University, she moved to Abilene, Texas, where she currently resides with her husband and five children. She recently co-authored the chapter "Transitioning a Simulation Center" with Michael Young in *Defining Excellence in Simulation Programs*. She has also been a simulation center design consultant.

Lindsey Scott, MSN, RN, began her career as an Emergency Medical Technician where she used her skills in the field of critical care. She received her BSN from York College of Pennsylvania and worked as a bedside nurse in the critical care unit. She later worked at Lancaster General Hospital in the Trauma-Neuro ICU where was able to participate in writing protocols and assisting in research. After moving to Austin, TX, Lindsey transitioned to position as a travel nurse in the ICU and pursued her Masters of Nursing with an emphasis in education through Grand Canyon University. Lindsey's most recent role was as a Program Coordinator with a Licensed Vocational Nursing department where she also helped with new simulation laboratories.

Emily Shaw, MA, CMI, EMT-B, has a decade of experience in simulation, which includes simulator development of the Virtual IV product line with Laerdal DC, providing education on scenario programming as Simulation Specialist for Laerdal Medical, and operating a simulation center for MedStar Health. Her current position is as the Northeast Territory Manager for Mimic Technologies, a pioneer in robotic surgery simulation. Her medical training started with combined post-baccalaureate and pre-med classes from Towson University and UMBC and the first year of medical school courses as part of the Johns Hopkins MA program. She completed her EMT-Basic certification in 2007 and her EMT-Paramedic program in 2011. Emily is a Certified Medical Illustrator with a Master of Arts degree in medical and biological illustration from Johns Hopkins Medical School; she also holds a Bachelor of Arts in fine art from Maryland Institute College of Art. In 2003 while at Hopkins, she was awarded a Vesalius Trust Alan W. Cole scholarship for her thesis project on trypanosome KDNA replication. For the past 14 years, she has been the sole proprietor of Illustrating Medicine (illustrating-medicine.com) with clients such as National Institutes of Health, Johnson & Johnson, and Lippincott Williams, & Wilkins. As an active member of the Society for Simulation in Healthcare (SSH), Emily volunteers with the SOTS Section as the Editor-in-Chief for the forthcoming Simulation Technology Operations and Resource Magazine which is to be published online quarterly by SSH. She also volunteers on the Hospital-Based Simulation Programs SIG having established their social media in 2014 including a Twitter feed: @SSH_HBSP. Emily gives back to her community by volunteering as an EMT-B at the Chestnut Ridge Volunteer Fire Company in Baltimore County, as well as serving on the Board of Governors for the Mount Washington Improvement Association. She remains active in the Association of Medical Illustrators by serving on the Board of Governors with the Executive Committee as Secretary, on the Sponsorship, Membership, PR Committees, and is the Twitter Editor of @AMIdotorg.

H. Michael Young, BBS, MDiv, CHSE, has worked within the healthcare simulation field over the last 9 years, first at Tarleton State University (TSU), and then for Level 3 Healthcare. In his role at TSU, Michael grew into a role best described as the simulation systems administrator, but like so many of those working in simulation operations, enjoyed the more generic title of Simulation Technology Specialist. As an active member of the Society for Simulation in Healthcare (SSH), Mr. Young served on the Board of Directors (2013) and the Accreditation Council. He currently serves as Chair of the SSH Certification Committee's subcommittee overseeing the *Certified Healthcare Simulation Operations Specialist* (CHSOS) professional certification. Mr. Young is also working on his doctorate (Ed.D.) at TSU in Educational Leadership with a core emphasis in Instructional Technology, and more specifically focused on healthcare simulation in education. In 2014, Mr. Young sought and received the Certified Healthcare Simulation Educator (CHSE) professional certification. Michael began work with Dr. Laura T. Gantt on this book in 2013.

ACKNOWLEDGMENTS

For his exceptional contributions to helping this book take flight, the editors would like to acknowledge John M. Rice, Chair, Government Relations Committee and Past Chair, Technology and Standards Committee for the Society for Simulation in Healthcare.

For her administrative and personal assistance with references and documents for this work, Laura T. Gantt would like to acknowledge Shelby L. Donnelly of East Carolina University College of Nursing.

For their responsiveness to eleventh hour calls for help, suggestions for reference material, and encouragement, we acknowledge the members of the Society for Simulation in Healthcare (SSH) and the International Nurses Association for Clinical Simulation and Learning (INACSL).

1

INTRODUCTION

Laura T. Gantt

East Carolina University College of Nursing, Greenville, NC, USA

Readers may recall the terms "digital native" and "digital immigrant" and the year(s) that they first became common vernacular. A digital native is typically one for whom technology has always existed; a digital immigrant, on the other hand, has migrated toward the use of technology out of necessity or a desire to integrate it into their lives (Prensky, 2001, p. 3). In this same way, it seems there are those of us who are simulation immigrants and others who are simulation natives. While I consider myself a native, I stop short of calling myself an expert. My background in emergency and flight nursing means that I have taken every type of certification course, many of which were "simulation based," long before they were called that. This gave me an unexpected edge in obtaining a position in the healthcare simulation field at a time when incredible financial resources were dedicated to developing simulation labs, even though few people knew much about them.

I did not, however, have an edge in finding the educational resources I needed to build a successful team of professionals for a simulation program in a large nursing college with diverse undergraduate and graduate degrees. Nevertheless, with limited resources, I set about the task of educating myself in healthcare simulation. At first, I attended simulator training and simulation conferences, and read the few books and journals available.

After a few years of blind searching, I got smarter in my hunt for resources. Indeed, in some fields of study, simulation really has been around a very long time. I looked at how other disciplines conducted simulation-based training. This proved to be helpful in determining best practices for teaching with simulation, since

Healthcare Simulation: A Guide for Operations Specialists, First Edition.
Edited by Laura T. Gantt and H. Michael Young.

other fields, such as aviation and gaming, have overlapping characteristics with healthcare.

However, when it came to training those who had to put it all together in the healthcare simulation lab, I learned the hard way that trying to apply lessons from other fields often does not work. Never was this clearer to me than when I encountered a new employee who could not learn the role or functions of the simulation operator or technologist in the lab. With previous employees, I guess I had been lucky enough to hire people with aptitudes for the work. However, for those who were inclined in the direction of technology, there were simply no journal articles, books, or guides to assist a person who might be struggling with assimilating the knowledge needed for this type of position. When I failed to find the information I needed to help my new hire, I was sure that I must not be looking in the right places yet. I was dismayed.

While I might have been distraught then, I was simultaneously elated and depressed to find that the problem I identified with a lack of resources for training simulation operators and technical staff had been previously well-described. As early as 1985, a National Research Council (NRC) report entitled Human Factors Aspects of Simulation (Jones, Hennessey, & Deutsch, 1985) outlined a number of issues, including the following:

- The number of personnel required to support simulators is substantial (p. 22).
- Difficulties in design and use of simulators could be reduced with analyses of the human skills and knowledge required for their operation and maintenance (p. 45).
- The human operator of a simulator may be able to compensate for simulator shortcomings, but this may result in negative transfer in training (p. 50).
- Activities of scenario generation and simulation control need to be described to permit understanding of functional flow (p. 65).

The types of simulators discussed by these authors include those used in aviation, motor vehicles, and nuclear power, but the above list could easily be applied today to patient simulators and those that operate them. While it may be argued that healthcare simulation has existed for several decades, resources have been slow to come along, particularly in the area of healthcare simulation technology. What the NRC wrote in 1985 was true then and, as often seems to be the case, little progress has been made in resolving simulation operator and technologist training across multiple fields.

To understand why the application of work from other fields that use simulation simply does not work when it comes to healthcare simulation may be, in part, because we do not yet fully know what it means exactly to be a simulation technologist or operations specialist. The position titles for this type of work vary wildly between organizations. The work itself involves knowing how to put human patient simulators together and troubleshoot them, how to network and program them, and how to operate them. While the human-to-machine interface is similar to other fields that use simulation, there is a difference with patient simulators that involves a relationship between living humans and patient simulators with a concurrent need for an understanding of proper patient care. In addition, simulation operations specialists (SOS), as I have come to call and know them, must also know what instructors and educators know about objectives and outcomes for varying levels and types of learners. They must know a good deal about the learners themselves and their roles; these learners may, at times, come from different disciplines and must, in the simulation lab and "in real life," work well together. While most aspects of patient simulation technology may be taught over time, other parts are "art" and require a talent for creativity and vision. A flare for the dramatic and the ability to write a script and then improvise from it are skills not usually associated with healthcare. But a simulation lab is much more than an arena for skills training. Many days, it is more like the production of a complicated play.

In 2013, the Society for Simulation in Healthcare (SSH) leadership voted to approve the name of a new certification for those working in the simulation operations arena: Certified Healthcare Simulation Operations Specialist (CHSOS). This certification was not designed for any one type of position, but is inclusive of many of the evolving roles within healthcare simulation. For the record, the planning and outline for this book predated the CHSOS and the book should not be assumed to be a preparatory book for the exam.

Also in 2013, SSH announced that "Sim Ops" would be the theme for the annual preconference symposium. Both the certification and the symposium are evidence that simulation operations are an important area of specialization within healthcare education, training, and assessment. There are two sides to *operations* in simulation programs: administration and execution. On the *administrative* side, *operations* refer to governance of simulation programs through policy, guidelines, and financials. On the *execution* side, *operations* refers to the implementation of tasks as defined by administration and subject matter experts.

For the purposes of this book, the SOS is someone who has advanced knowledge and understanding of the many facets of day-to-day operations within a healthcare simulation lab. Because educators tend to be technologically challenged, the SOS usually has a technology background, but must also be part educator, part engineer, part director, and part artist. The resources that we have at our disposal to train SOS in any of the required realms are slim to none. The titles for the chapters in this book occurred to me over the course of an average month in the clinical simulation laboratory. For example, consider Chapter 8, which is about the fit between the employer and potential SOS. The chapter was originally entitled, "Just Call Me Gumby." On a routine day in the simulation lab, those who bring the action to life are truly stretched into any number of positions, some flattering and others more compromising. "Sure, just call me Gumby" is the likely response to a faculty or staff question that begins with "Can't you just………………………" Typically, this blank is filled in by the requestor with something like "fix this?" or "take care of that?" or "help this student?" or "relocate that class and/or piece of equipment?"

The purpose of this book is to help people who specialize in simulation operations figure out how to get started. The book begins with chapters on the current state of the simulation professional workforce and how it has evolved. From there the book moves through topics of interest to those in the simulation workforce related to the art, science, and innovation necessary for the role of the SOS.

Each of the chapter authors for this book was recruited not because they needed to share how to do a job, but because of the innovative work that they have done to develop the role of the SOS. There are a few "how to" simulation books already available. The focus of those has been the educator or instructor role in simulation or simulation center development and leadership. In this book, however, each author was asked to address a topic of interest, some from novice and others from expert perspectives, in which they truly are specialists of the highest degree. Each of these authors has become indispensable because they are doing groundbreaking work that perhaps no one else has even thought of, much less done. The types of simulation professionals who discuss their work in this book have become crucial to the work of healthcare educators and researchers alike.

One colleague of mine feels certain that the day is rapidly coming when those of us at the helms of simulation centers will become unnecessary and obsolete. We were the ones that got the simulators out of the boxes, got everything running, and figured out how to make it all work in the beginning. But we are not the future of healthcare simulation. Our protégés, whether they are educators, engineers, technologists, or managers, have outperformed us and taken it to another level that involves increasing amounts of technical knowledge, creativity, and innovation. They were out of the boxes before the simulators were. For those of us who helped get simulation started in healthcare, our collective job now is to help healthcare simulation progress from its current status by making sure that the next generation comes along with a bigger toolbox than we had.

REFERENCES

Jones, E. R., Hennessey, R. T., & Deutsch, S. (1985). *Human factors aspects of simulation.* Washington, DC: National Academy Press.

Prensky, M. (2001). Digital natives, digital immigrants: Part 1. *On the Horizon, 9*(5), 1–6. 10.1108/10748120110424816

2

HEALTHCARE SIMULATION OPERATIONS: BRIDGING THE GAPS

H. MICHAEL YOUNG

Level 3 Healthcare, Mesa, AZ, USA

INTRODUCTION

Use of simulation in healthcare has become pervasive within undergraduate clinical and pre-hospital education, hospital continuing education programs, and in various medical school specialties. Often, clinical and medical faculty are responsible for the day-to-day operations of many simulation programs, typically in addition to their other responsibilities. Today, simulation operations is not just the domain of educators and program administrators, but also of various specialists, with different titles, roles, and responsibilities. A small simulation program will be fortunate to have one full-time staff member, regardless of specialty, but larger programs will have diverse teams of specialists, especially those working in simulation operations. Nevertheless, simulation operations is still relatively new to many simulation programs that have long held the opinion that operations is the domain of administration. The technology that has emerged within the simulation program has become very sophisticated and complex thus can benefit from the utilization of expertise from a diverse group of professionals, including those inside and outside of the healthcare domain (Alinier, Pozzo, & Shields, 2008; Gantt, 2012, p. 580). The simulation community, in general, has grown and expanded because of enterprising clinical educators who took the lead as early adopters in the use of these simulation technologies known commonly as "patient simulators." Simulation has long been a part of clinical education, but the advancing complexity and interoperability of today's technology has advanced a

Healthcare Simulation: A Guide for Operations Specialists, First Edition.
Edited by Laura T. Gantt and H. Michael Young.
© 2016 John Wiley & Sons, Inc. Published 2016 by John Wiley & Sons, Inc.

meaningful dialogue about specialized staffing and a need for a broader system perspective (Jones, Hennessy, & Deutsch, 1985, p. 86). Early adopters comprised the initial simulation operations team, and many of these innovators still serve as the first line of support for their respective programs. Recruitment of the simulation operations specialist (SOS) draws primarily from a pool of RNs, EMTs, allied health, and IT professionals (Foster, Sheriff, & Cheney, 2008, p. 141; Society for Simulation in Healthcare [SSH], 2013, p. 10; Vollmer, Mönk, & Heinrichs, 2008, p. 628; Zigmont, Oocumma, Szyld, & Maestre, 2015, p. 551). However, educator workload has often necessitated the creation of additional operational roles. Such roles may include, but are not limited to, *simulation technician, simulation specialist, simulation technology specialist, simulation operator,* and others (Education Advisory Board [EAB], 2013, p. 25), as well as non-simulation specific roles. Thanks to the introduction of SSH's *Certified Healthcare Simulation Operations Specialist* (CHSOS); these roles, and others, are now being organized into a new class of specialist now referred to as the *SOS*. As simulation technologies continue to become more sophisticated and interoperable, so too has the demand for more specialized staff who have strong backgrounds in information technology (IT), audiovisual (AV) technology, project management, and engineering. Such personnel work alongside their clinical counterparts in their simulation programs and are responsible for coordinating the preparation, maintenance, and implementation of healthcare simulation, also known as *simulation operations*.

Why Is Simulation Operations Emerging as a Specialty?

New professional roles are emerging as the result of the identification of *gaps* in the simulation program's ability to address the demands in clinical and medical education. Such gaps include (i) the rising shortage of faculty (American Association of Colleges of Nursing [AACN], 2015), (ii) increasing demands on the *time* of faculty, and (iii) a growing need for specialized knowledge, skills, and attributes (or *KSAs*). The latter relates to the issues around multiple layers of technological systems that must work together; this requires additional expertise, or the sharing of task responsibilities with one or more SOSs in order to achieve both immediate and long-term goals of simulation operations. This chapter will first identify many of the "gaps" emerging out of simulation operations, in general, and suggest ways in which such gaps are "bridged" with the emerging roles now identified as SOSs. "Gaps" in simulation programs can be defined as those recurring challenges that fall outside the expertise of the simulation team members, whether faculty or staff. By distributing tasks among specialized support staff, such as the SOS, subject matter experts are free to focus on those tasks for which they are uniquely qualified.

GAP #1: TECHNOLOGICAL EXPERTISE

SOSs, in general, have made the task of setting up and operating simulators easier for busy fulltime simulation educators and program faculty, freeing them to focus on the scenario design and participant assessment rather than operational logistics. Despite the emergence of the various SOS roles, the technical demands of a simulation program *may* still exceed the expertise of existing staff (Vollmer et al., 2008, p. 628).

In general, when technological systems fail, who provides *timely* support (Dieckmann, Lippert, Glavin, & Rall, 2010, pp. 219–220)? Typically, institutional IT departments may pass this burden on to the vendor, while others would say that the IT department should help solve the problem. With technical delays comes a delay in resolution, and with the delay in resolution comes delays in scheduled activities and loss of operational efficiency. When a simulation system component fails during a scenario, an extended warranty is of little help when it requires that the simulator be repaired somewhere else in the world at a vendor support center. Unless the implementation of backup plan has been planned or resources are on hand (Dieckmann et al., 2010, p. 220), the scheduled educational event must be cancelled or rescheduled (Canales & Huang, 2015). The healthcare simulation community has relied heavily on vendor provided extended warranties for ongoing technical support. However, while critical to the simulation program's sustainability, warranties alone are not an adequate solution. Even if the simulator does not need to be shipped elsewhere for repair, vendor phone support can be time-consuming, and neither the caller nor the support person may be able to clearly communicate cause and effect (LaCombe & Whiteside, 2015, p. 341). Hence, a simulation program likely needs an SOS who is specifically trained and experienced in IT to overcome support issues that are the result of multiple system interoperability (e.g. network and simulator) (Vollmer et al., 2008, p. 633). For additional information on these systems, the reader is referred to Chapter 9.

GAP #2: TRAINING

Just as an RN or EMT new to simulation must receive training to use specialized technologies outside their experience (e.g. simulators), so must an IT or AV specialist learn the language and concepts related to human physiology, medical terminology and concepts, especially as it relates to the scope of capability of the simulators being used. The questions then becomes, what form will this training take? Who is qualified to teach it? Training programs for simulation professionals are typically designed for clinicians/educators working in academic or hospital environments. These persons managed all aspects of simulator adoption and utilization within the last 10–15 years. However, these training curricula fail to take into account the current trend toward the possibility that an SOS trainee could be someone who does *not* come from a medical or clinical background; hence, the potential for bringing in technical expertise from non-healthcare sectors is reduced because such candidates are not even considered for an SOS role. There is evidence that the need for non-clinician and IT simulation training is expanding (Griffin-Sobel et al., 2010).

Funding the Right Priorities for Training

Program administrators, through adequately funded training mandates, must be called upon to develop the scope and priority of a comprehensive training initiative. Local, regional, national, and international opportunities for continuing education in healthcare simulation are abundant. However, when educators and technical staff are expected to use only personal funds to attend, training is unlikely to occur. When programs do not invest, the probability that individuals will pay their own way is unlikely. A shift in priorities related to budgetary planning is required to ensure that simulation expertise can keep pace with the rate of simulation technology adoption. Training is necessary for both simulation program staff and institutional IT leadership who need key knowledge and skills to support a developing, robust education program.

GAP #3: DIVISION OF LABOR

Educators/Clinicians: The simulation operations team is best understood in the context of the entire simulation team, not just one particular role (Griffin-Sobel et al., 2010, pp. 41–43). Some simulation programs have the benefit of clinical educators who were early adopters and then became the primary simulation technology experts out of necessity. However, as simulation has become more technologically sophisticated and complex, expectations have changed. Support of one or two simulators utilized in a skills lab has, in many programs, progressed to over a dozen or more advanced simulators in dedicated simulation labs, with one or more control rooms and an integrated audiovisual system. Simulation technology systems include components manufactured and configured by many different vendors, each with their own proprietary system requirements and features. As a result, clinical simulation specialists, whether they are operations specialists or faculty, are learning that it is not easy to decipher whom to call when a particular part of the system fails to operate correctly (See LaCombe & Whiteside, 2015, pp. 340–342 for tips). For example, some simulators communicate with the control computer wirelessly, but do not utilize the local network. Other simulators depend on the local network (wired or wireless). One type of system depends on proprietary methods of connection, and other simulators rely on ubiquitous technologies supported by institutional IT departments. Many simulation professionals will likely not know the difference without years of practical experience. The emergence of the SOS role allows for greater diversity within the operations team, and thus frees the clinical educator to focus on issues related to their role as subject matter experts. However, reliance on other subject matter experts in the field of technology is a growing, acceptable—and in many circumstances—necessary approach to bridge gaps in knowledge and attributes of the overall simulation operations team.

Technicians/Technologists: The label of "tech" or "technician" has developed some negative connotations in simulation circles, according to the CHSOS Job Analysis team. During the development of the CHSOS, the job analysis team explored a number of names for the new professional certification. While some of the "technicians" had no problem with the designation, most preferred other titles. Two reasons were cited by those simulation technicians present: (i) technicians in hospitals are entry level roles and (ii) hospital technician roles would almost certainly result in lower pay. The perception exists that many in those roles do not prefer the title "simulation technician." Some simulation programs have preferred the title "simulation technology specialist" (STS) in large part due to the work of the DACUM Competency Profile developed by a California Community Colleges group (California Community College Economic and Workforce Development Program Health Initiative [RHORC/HCI], 2008). In August 2014, SimGHOSTS voted to adopt the STS designation as a preferred title. However, due to influence of the CHSOS professional certification, some programs have begun using the title *SOS* for their operations staff, thus avoiding the term "technician" altogether. Regardless of what the position is titled, or the precise meaning attributed to the word "technician," the employment of such specialists as *SOSs* can be a critical part of the simulation operations team, thus bridging gaps with the knowledge, skills, and attributes not present in other SOS or educator roles.

For those simulation program administrators tasked with hiring the SOS, two professional backgrounds are preferred in their candidates, with the greater of the two being the first:

1. Experience in the healthcare professional community (such as an RN or EMT).
2. Comfort with technology, usually specific to personal computers or audiovisual equipment (See Chapter 8).

Having both backgrounds (healthcare, technology) represented is critical to the success of any simulation program. Since such backgrounds are typically difficult to find in one candidate, consideration of hiring specialists that are strong in IT to work alongside clinical staff could provide the desired synergy. Where the RN or EMT may lack the required competency related to technology, the IT specialist is strong. Where the IT specialist is less knowledgeable about healthcare and human anatomy/physiology, the RN or EMT are trained. Together, their skills can coalesce and provide needed flexibility and redundancy, reducing downtime and encouraging innovation. When considering candidates, maintaining an open mind to hiring from different backgrounds is necessary. Technology is pervasive across many fields, including multimedia production, engineering, informatics, instructional technology, and fine arts. The various SOS roles have the potential to be rich in professional diversity.

Managers and Administrators: Like many specialist roles, *it takes one to know one*. A common problem with many simulation program administrators and educators is that they often do not have *advanced* technical knowledge and skills that they would otherwise require of their specialists. Consequently, decision-makers then have to assess technological skills primarily on the assertions of the candidate's self-assessment of their technical capabilities. Talking "tech" is not difficult in today's culture where so many work with it daily. Anyone considering a candidate for a job as an SOS must recognize that people are consumers of technology, and rarely have more than a peripheral knowledge of the words and concepts used in conversations. To develop a strong simulation operations workforce that truly reflects technical expertise, simulation program leadership should invite hospital or university IT managers to participate in candidate interviews. Simulation program management can then determine how the candidate's temperament and teamwork skills will fit within the program. Involving IT management or hiring an IT consultant during the hiring process can also help win the institutional IT department's support in giving new hires access to network and server resources; such resources will help with simulation technology integration, function, and innovation.

GAP #4: COMMON LANGUAGE AND CULTURE

The reasons why RNs, EMTs, and allied health professionals are often preferred for simulation operations roles within healthcare simulation programs is primarily because of the knowledge, language, and culture. However, the biggest obstacle to learning either the clinical or the technological side of the job is not necessarily the same for any two candidates from either domain. The biggest challenge to the IT-oriented SOS is not so much the language as it is the breadth of the professional healthcare culture. This is the same problem clinicians have when trying to learn and do tasks typically attributed to IT professionals. Navigating the technical manuals, helpdesk personnel, and various special domains within the IT industry takes different but equal amounts of skill and cultural awareness. The balance of technical or clinical SOS team members a simulation program will need depends largely on the program objectives and individuals that are hired. Many simulation programs do not have the benefit of support roles such as the SOS, but the role is becoming critical. If only one SOS can be hired, it is all the more important that the SOS be strong in IT. See also Chapter 9 for *Foundations of the Simulation Operations Specialist*.

GAP #5: MISUNDERSTOOD IT

A common misunderstanding within many institutions is that the IT department is one entity within an organization. Just as it takes a variety of healthcare specialists to meet the needs of staff and clients, so is the case for the IT industry. IT consists of various departments and divisions, each with their own specialties and organizational hierarchy. The SOS should be as aware of these IT divisions as they are of the simulation technologies they maintain and operate.

The responsibility of an institution's IT team includes the management of network security, computers, servers, and user credentials (logins and permissions). At times, the end users' perception of the IT professional is that they are more concerned about what the end user should NOT do, rather than what might be possible. Despite any perceptions from those they serve, IT has to be concerned with preventing problems as much as solving new problems. The objectives of a simulation program may be in conflict with the policies of an IT department, especially as it relates to the infrastructure of the institution. Chapter 9 discusses the language and concepts common among IT professionals, and terminology that a SOS would benefit from knowing.

IT may not assign personnel to address ongoing operational and technological challenges common to simulation programs. If IT leadership do not understand the simulation program's needs or technology it uses, roadblocks to support will likely emerge. Simulation program administrators, educators, and SOSs must be persistent in clarifying support needs to IT leadership (Kim, Hewitt, Buis, & Ross, 2015, p. 71).

MINDING THE GAPS AND IDENTIFYING SOLUTIONS

First, as previously discussed, simulation technology *is* instructional technology and can potentially draw from underutilized resources. Second, the need to diversify the role of the SOS by employing a mix of technical *and* clinical experts will encourage innovation. Other considerations for minding the "gaps" would be to find the right person for the job, encourage and support continuing education.

The Right Fit

When considering who will be operating the simulators, the decision on who to hire will depend on how scenarios are routinely operated, and if the subject matter expert is present in the control room during those scenarios (see Chapters 10 and 11). If the educator is sitting at the operator's side, providing direction during the scenario, then having a clinician at the controls is not critical. Familiarity and capability of interacting with the control software is the primary concern. However, if the operators *are* responsible for directing the outcomes of the scenario without an appropriate subject matter expert present, then having an experienced healthcare provider would be the better choice. Such personnel, with appropriate training, can also facilitate the debriefing since they may have been in a position to observe the student participants while also operating the simulator. One of the reasons many simulation centers run scenarios "on-the-fly" is that the process of programming a scenario is time consuming and requires a high degree of technical comfort. An AV technician can certainly operate a patient simulator, but this may not be the best use of such a professional. This person should not operate the simulator without some explicit direction from an experienced clinical or medical educator. An alternative to having a subject matter expert present at the time of the simulation operation is the use of validated, well-programmed (automated) scenarios. Chapter 10 discusses this in length.

Continuing Education

To address many of the previously identified gaps, the technical workforce must continue to evolve in its development. At the International Meeting for Simulation in Healthcare (IMSH) 2012, the Society for Simulation in Healthcare recruited *technicians* to develop a curriculum and recruit subject matter experts for nearly two dozen technical sessions intended to orient technicians new in their roles. However, many of the attendees in these sessions were clinical educators and coordinators in their respective programs who also wanted a more practical understanding of the tools they were using. As mentioned earlier, the Society for Simulation in Healthcare has developed a certification program for SOSs (technicians). The International Nursing Association for Clinical Simulation and Learning (INACSL) has also seen the need for developing operations and technology content, and offers sessions suited for nursing educators and non-educators who need to expand their technical expertise. Smaller nursing simulation programs with tighter budgets may benefit from the INACSL conference's affordability. Opportunities for development of the SOS team benefits the entire simulation team, as each SOS is tasked with using simulation technology at one level or another.

Vendor-Provided Training

Vendors continue to provide entry-level training for the simulators they sell. In recent years, though, expanded technical training, including mannequin repair, has become available to some operations specialists. Many educators expect plug and play operation from these simulation technologies, and are frustrated when they begin to understand the true technical demands of simulation. This makes it all the more important for a simulation program to send an SOS to these advanced courses so they can better support the educators in their programs.

CONCLUSION

Simulation is at a critical point in its development. An evaluation and strategy is needed for simulation program staffing and workforce development. Whether a simulation program is hospital-based, academic, or stand-alone, interprofessional collaboration and communication among simulation operations team members is important. Simulation program educators and administrators must cultivate expertise beyond the ranks of clinicians/educators to fill simulation staffing and distributed roles successfully. The simulation operations team would benefit from a common language, knowledge, and cultural values, regardless of the professional domain, education type, or experience of each team member.

Simulation in healthcare education is still quite young, having moved out of its infancy and now is in the midst of its adolescence over the last decade. To reach maturity, simulation operations as a field of expertise must be embraced as an opportunity to move beyond theory to find technological solutions and innovation.

As early as 1985, experts in U.S. government simulation practice state that simulators tend not to be used properly. Their words ring true for many in healthcare simulation:

> Some components that contribute to quality of use are scenarios, training techniques, operating and test procedures, instructor and operator knowledge and skills, proficiency assessment methods, and support features such as properly designed control consoles .... This process requires considerable specialized effort and, for cost reasons and lack of appreciation of its ultimate importance, is often neglected. (Jones et al., 1985, p. 93)

This book offers various perspectives on the role of the SOS, and to some extent the SOS' role in being a part of that "specialized effort." The following chapters demonstrate the scope and breadth of simulation operations as embodied in the specialist. Regardless of the title or specialization, members of the simulation operations team will empower educators and researchers to prepare future generations of practitioners to improve patient outcomes.

REFERENCES

Alinier, G., Pozzo, R., & Shields, C. (2008). Hybrid vigor: The simulation professional. In R. R. Kyle, Jr. & W. B. Murray (Eds.), *Clinical simulation: Operations, engineering and management* (pp. 505–506). London: Elsevier.

American Association of Colleges of Nursing. (2015). *Nursing faculty shortage fact sheet* [Fact sheet]. Retrieved August 7, 2015, from http://www.aacn.nche.edu/media-relations/FacultyShortageFS.pdf

California Community College Economic and Workforce Development Program Health Initiative. (2008). *DACUM competency profile for simulation technology specialist.* Retrieved August 7, 2015, from http://ca-hwi.org/files/dacums/Simulation%20Technology%20 Specialist-FINAL.doc

Canales, C., & Huang, Y. M. (2015). Expecting the unexpected: Contingency planning for healthcare simulation. In J. C. Palaganas, J. C. Maxworthy, C. A. Epps, & M. E. Mancini (Eds.), *Defining excellence in simulation programs* (pp. 582–591). Hong Kong: Wolters Kluwer.

Dieckmann, P., Lippert, A., Glavin, R., & Rall, M. (2010, August). When things do not go as expected: scenario life savers. *Simulation in Healthcare, 5*(4), 219–225.

Education Advisory Board. (2013). *Considerations for online medical simulation technician training programs.* Retrieved June 24, 2015, from Education Advisory Board website http://www.eab.com/research-and-insights/continuing-and-online-education-forum/custom/2013/12/considerations-for-online-medical-simulation-technician-training-programs

Foster, J. G., Sheriff, S., & Cheney, S. (2008, May/June). Using nonfaculty registered nurses to facilitate high-fidelity human patient simulation activities. *Nurse Educator, 33*(3), 137–141.

Gantt, L. (2012, November). Who's driving? the role and training of the human patient simulation operator. *CIN: Computers, Informatics, Nursing, 30*, 579–586.

Griffin-Sobel, J. P., Acee, A., Sharoff, L., Cobus-Kuo, L., Woodstock-Wallace, A., & Dornbaum, M. (2010, January). A transdisciplinary approach to faculty development. Nursing education technology. *Nursing Education Perspectives, 31*(1), 41–43.

Jones, E. R., Hennessy, R. T., & Deutsch, S. (Eds.). (1985). *Human factors aspects of simulation.* Washington, DC: National Academy Press. Retrieved June 24, 2015, from https://books.google.com/books?id=KEErAAAAYAAJ&printsec=frontcover&source=gbs_ge_summary_r&cad=0#v=onepage&q&f=false

Kim, S., Hewitt, W., Buis, J. A., & Ross, B. K. (2015). Creating the infrastructure for a successful simulation program. In J. C. Palaganas, J. C. Maxworthy, C. A. Epps, & M. E. Mancini (Eds.), *Defining excellence in simulation programs* (pp. 66–89). Hong Kong: Wolters Kluwer.

LaCombe, D. M., & Whiteside, G. (2015). Working with vendors. In J. C. Palaganas, J. C. Maxworthy, C. A. Epps, & M. E. Mancini (Eds.), *Defining excellence in simulation programs* (pp. 334–344). Hong Kong: Wolters Kluwer.

Society for Simulation in Healthcare. (2013). *Certified healthcare simulation operations specialist: Job analysis demographics and results summary*. Retrieved June 24, 2015, from www.ssih.org: http://www.ssih.org

Vollmer, J., Mönk, S., & Heinrichs, W. (2008). Staff education for simulation: Train-the-trainer concepts. In R. R. Kyle, Jr. & W. B. Murray (Eds.), *Clinical simulation: Operations, engineering and management* (pp. 625–642). London: Elsevier.

Zigmont, J., Oocumma, N., Szyld, D., & Maestre, J. M. (2015). Educator training and simulation methodology courses. In J. C. Palaganas, J. C. Maxworthy, C. A. Epps, & M. E. Mancini (Eds.), *Defining excellence in simulation programs* (pp. 546–557). Hong Kong: Wolters Kluwer.

3

EVOLUTION OF THE SIMULATION OPERATIONS SPECIALIST (SOS)

JESIKA S. GAVILANES
Oregon Health & Science University, Portland, OR, USA

BRIEF HISTORY OF THE EVOLUTION OF SIMULATION IN HEALTHCARE

Simulation has played an integral role in training multiple disciplines for decades (Rosen, 2008). As the healthcare system has increased in complexity, so has the evolution of the role of the simulation operations specialist (SOS) within simulation and healthcare.

Historically, there was not a specific school or training track for an SOS to gain the needed skills, knowledge, and abilities for this role. People came to simulation operations almost randomly, some with computer and technology background, others from an audio and video and classroom support background, and many from various clinical backgrounds. Some operations specialists came from EMT, RN, and other allied health fields. As early as 2006, some expressed a desire to see the simulation technician role as a professional career track (Michael Young, personal oral communication, May 8, 2015). Gantt (2012, p. 579) stated in an article that "little can be found in the literature about the role, educational background, or training of the simulation operator." She (2012) also explored the roles and variations between operators and technicians.

As simulation technology has advanced, the expectations placed on the SOS have also grown. A history of simulation in healthcare is outlined in *The Comprehensive Textbook of Healthcare Simulation* (Levine, DeMaria, Schwartz, & Sim, 2014).

Healthcare Simulation: A Guide for Operations Specialists, First Edition.
Edited by Laura T. Gantt and H. Michael Young.
© 2016 John Wiley & Sons, Inc. Published 2016 by John Wiley & Sons, Inc.

Since the early implications of Dr. Abrahamson's creation of the Sim1 in 1964, there has been continuous expansion of simulation technologies (Rosen, 2008). Along with this technical evolution, there was also a growing need to increase capacity for simulation experiences within school systems and hospitals. With increased student enrollment and more expansive healthcare education facilities, some visionaries started to acknowledge the need for a professional career track for individuals in the SOS role. Although some early adopters may have shared this thinking, the majority did not. Until 2012, there was no documented or "official" interest.

In response to a Society for Simulation in Healthcare SH Sim Connect survey, various contributors shared their experiences of their early days of simulation integration. The responses came from simulation facilities across the United States and Canada. Challenges to hiring a dedicated SOS were connected to issues of funding and lack of executive buy-in (Kim Baily, personal email communication, April 30, 2015).

Colette Foisy-Doll with Robbins Health Learning Center in Canada first got involved with simulation operations in 1998. She was asked to be a full-time faculty running a lab that utilized low-to high-fidelity simulation. This was the first such a position that Foisy-Doll was aware of in nursing undergraduate programs in Canada. Foisy-Doll shared that it was by 2007 that they first had a 0.5 full-time equivalent (FTE) allocated to simulation technology and that they hired their first full-time simulation technologist in 2011 (Colette Foisy-Doll, personal email communication, April 30, 2015). Benny Holland shared that in 2005, "I had never received any of my education through simulation technology, but I started opening boxes and hooking up simulators" (Benny Holland, personal email communication, April 30, 2015).

In 2003, the Oregon Health & Science University (OHSU) hired both a dedicated Master's prepared nurse educator and a simulation technician (at the time her working title was as a media coordinator) to administer the simulation operations in their program. The simulation technician did not come from a healthcare background, but rather was flexible, great with technology, extremely organized, a clear communicator, and able to create realistic simulation environments. The OHSU simulation team was comprised of just the two professionals at that time. Since those early days, OHSU has evolved into a 20,000 square foot facility with eight full-time simulation operations team members. Their titles vary depending on the focus of their position. Positions that are represented are as follows:

- Simulation Technology Specialist, Program Tech I,
- Simulation Operations Specialist, Program Tech II,
- Clinical Education Specialist (Program Tech II working with clinical units in the hospital with simulation/educational research and teaching ACLS),
- Clinical Skills Program Coordinator, Project Coordinator,
- Standardized Patient Program Coordinator, Project Coordinator,
- Standardized Patient Program Technician, Program Tech I,
- Director of Operations/Operations Manager, Program Administrator III.

Within the OHSU programs, various manikins and features for different models have been utilized in multiple types of environments used for simulation sessions. For example, at OHSU in Portland Oregon, there are eight simulation theaters that can be set up to recreate a(n):

- medical surgical environment(s),
- home health setting,
- intensive care unit,
- emergency room/trauma bay,
- operating room,
- labor and delivery room,
- pediatric intensive care unit,
- post-anesthesia care unit.

The significance of this is that the SOS needs to be able to assist the faculty and clinical experts with improved realism in these various settings, as well as appropriately utilize the technologies available in the facility.

In speaking with a current SOS whose working job title is clinical skills program coordinator, Trenell Croskey shared that he was in school for psychology when he fell into simulation operations. He has now been in simulation for 3 years and currently works at the OHSU Simulation Center at the Collaborative Life Science Building (CLSB). Previously he was not working directly in patient care, but was working in the hospital. He had experience as an administrative coordinator and that was why he was hired for the simulation center. Most of the simulation operations aspects of his job were learned through on-the-job training and that these grew over time. He felt his "can-do" attitude made him versatile and open to learning and doing whatever it takes to get a job done. He feels simulation is more than operating the simulators and states:

> You have to think of how each group is using simulation skills, using a high-fidelity manikin, and what are their goals. Being able to roll with anything and being solution-oriented is essential to this role. You never know when something is going to work. You may test something and pause it and then when you get back it doesn't work. So, being able to stay calm on the outside is key. (Trenell Croskey, personal oral communication, May 11, 2015)

Lish Robinson shared that she first got involved with simulation in 2006 when she was an anesthesia residency coordinator. She returned to working full-time in simulation in 2012 and says she likes it because she enjoys "watching people suddenly understand something visually" (Lish Robinson, personal oral communication, May 12, 2015).

INCREASING NEED FOR SIMULATION OPERATIONS SPECIALISTS

The need for a dedicated SOS became clearer in 2008 with the publishing of the first book on simulation operations, *Clinical Simulation: Operations, Engineering and Management* (Kyle & Murray, 2008). Throughout this "Big Green Book" (as it has come to be known), authors shared their perspectives on the growing need for a dedicated SOS. Hwang and Bencken (2008, p. 237) describe the "importance to have at least one part time technical support person." Stern (2008, p. 209) describes the various simulators and the need for an operator. Stern goes on to justify this need based on the need for "regular updating, cleaning, maintenance, expendable parts replacement, and repair; the staffing and employment requirements to meet these responsibilities are a major expense in treasure for finding, teaching, and retaining them." Michael C. Foss (2008a, p. 232) states: "At least two full-time laboratory technicians are needed to operate at the capacity needed for hundreds of students on and off campus, and thousands of patient events." Guillaume Alinier (2008, p. 270) goes on to expand on the simulation suite and that in the ideal world one simulation technician would be assigned to each simulation "stage" depending on space and utilization demands.

THE SOS IN THE BEGINNING

Certainly, in the beginning, a strong focus was on the technological skills aspects of the roles now associated with that of the SOS. With the increased adoption rate of high-fidelity patient simulators, an immediate need for technical expertise was identified in order to address all of the complexities of evolving simulation technologies. Maran and Glavin, in a 2003 publication, began to describe and evaluate the growing number of simulation training tools and manikins available on the market, including each product's various functions. Jeffries (2005) describes the role of the simulation operator as part of the student support component within simulation design.

The first operations specialists were educators. As early adopters, educators also maintained and operated the simulators. However, as simulation technologies became more complex and the educator's workload demands increased, the need for expanding the simulation team was described as necessary (Foss, 2008b, p. 232). The SOS emerged to partner with clinical experts to provide adequate support in order for simulation sessions to be successful. Based on the added complexities of more advanced manikins, live audio and video streaming of the simulations, recording and playback, an SOS now also needs to understand computers, networks, and AV systems.

MORE THAN SIMULATORS

Many early adopters in the simulation world were well aware of simulation as a teaching modality. In the beginning, the primary role of the SOS was to run the simulation manikin. In reality, the role of the SOS was and continues to be much more complicated, which emphasizes that the SOS is an essential member of the operations team in moving toward more effective simulation experiences. For example, the SOS functions at times as artist, producer, director, and conductor (see Chapter 5). This includes the integration and partnership with standardized patients (SPs) and other participants. Some SOS professionals work with faculty on the requested demographics of an actor or SP as described in their template or script. Although it may not be "typical," some simulation programs utilize the SOS to schedule the actors to come and play the part of the family members or the patient in the simulation theater. However, Objective Structured Clinical Examination (OSCE) centers with a dedicated SP program will often have a SP program coordinator who is also a part of the simulation operations team. The SP program coordinator and SP program technician interface directly with the faculty to ensure the actors are scheduled and available for the needed scenarios. Regardless of the scheduling task responsibilities, once the actor or SP arrives on site, the SOS may work with the actor to get them in place before the start of a scenario.

PAST AND PRESENT TRAINING OPPORTUNITIES

In the early 2000s, academic institution simulation programs across the country deliberately facilitated simulation technician training events. In 2006, there was a Tech Training conducted by Dean Michael C. Foss and Director of Education Patricia Hanrahan from the Springfield Technical Community College (STCC). The training was held at the SIMS Medical Center—A Virtual Hospital @ STCC. Three SOS leaders and educators from the Oregon Simulation Alliance spent 3 days learning from this team about their perspectives on the role of the SOS and the technical training needed. The Oregon Simulation Alliance also taught simulation technology curricula regionally to individuals from Washington State, Oregon, California, and Idaho. From 2006 to 2015, over 100 simulation technologists were trained across the region by attending the 2–3 day Simulation Technology Academy.

In 2011, Lance Baily founded The Gathering of Technicians, or GOT SIM, which eventually was renamed SimGHOSTS or "The Gathering of Healthcare Simulation Technology Specialists." This was the first professional development organization dedicated to the roles of the operations specialists.

In 2012, the Society for Simulation in Healthcare (SSH) moved toward incorporating technical content in their IMSH programming. Consequently, H. Michael Young was asked to chair a task group made up of SOSs for the purpose of defining topics and recruiting appropriate presenters from the operations specialist community. The technical content was very popular for both educators and those in technical operations. In November of 2012, SSH president-elect Paul Phrampus recruited Young to a 1-year appointment on the SSH Board of Directors. The success of the 2013 technical content sessions encouraged IMSH leadership to make even more technical content available in 2014. Consequently, IMSH 2014 hosted a simulation operations pre-conference in San Francisco where about 300 attendees participated in sessions and plenaries addressing administrative, technical, and operational issues and trends. H. Michael Young (personal oral communication, May 8, 2015) shared that he thought Dr. Phrampus was responding to what he felt was an underrepresented, yet essential, group within simulation operations. Young states that "there was a strong cry for 'Sim Techs' to have a certification to provide validity in the overall field of simulation."

In July 2014, a second SSH-sponsored simulation operations conference was hosted by the Peter M. Winter Institute for Simulation Education and Research (WISER) in Pittsburg, also with about 300 people in attendance. To date, SSH has not sponsored events for SOSs beyond the annual IMSH meeting. Clearly, at this point, IMSH session content has become an attractive resource for those interested in simulation operations and technology and those geared toward SOS goals and needs. SOSs have a dedicated content track at the International Meeting for Simulation in Healthcare (IMSH) in addition to education and research topics. As with any profession, there is a need for ongoing continuing education and networking.

REFERENCES

Alinier, G. (2008). The patient simulation suite. In R. R. Kyle & W. B. Murray (Eds.), *Clinical simulation: Operations, engineering, and management*. Burlington, MA: Elsevier.

Foss, M. C. (2008a). Retrofitting existing space for patient simulation. In R. R. Kyle & W. B. Murray (Eds.), *Clinical simulation: Operations, engineering, and management*. Burlington, MA: Elsevier.

Foss, M. C. (2008b). The nest form follows the essential functions. In R. R. Kyle & W. B. Murray (Eds.), *Clinical simulation: Operations, engineering, and management*. Burlington, MA: Elsevier.

Gantt, L. (2012). Who's driving? The role and training of the human patient simulation operator. *CIN: Computers, Informatics, Nursing, 30*(11), 579–586.

Hwang, J. C. F., & Bencken, B. (2008). Integrating simulation with existing clinical educational programs. In R. R. Kyle & W. B. Murray (Eds.), *Clinical simulation: Operations, engineering, and management*. Burlington, MA: Elsevier.

Jeffries, P. R. (2005). A framework for designing, implementing, and evaluating simulations used as teaching strategies in nursing. *Nursing Education Perspectives, 26*(2), 96–103.

Kyle, R. R., & Murray, W. B. (2008) *Clinical simulation: Operations, engineering, and management*. Burlington, MA: Elsevier.

Levine, A. I. DeMaria, S., Schwartz, A. D., & Sim, A. J. (2014). *The comprehensive textbook of medical simulation*. New York: Springer.

Maran, N. J., & Glavin, R. J. (2003). Low—to high—fidelity simulation—a continuum of medical education? *Medical Education, 37*(s1), 22–28.

Rosen, K. R. (2008). The history of medical simulation. *Journal of Critical Care, 23*, 157–166.

Stern, D. H. (2008). Choosing full-function patient simulators, creating and using the simulation suite. In R. R. Kyle & W. B. Murray (Eds.), *Clinical simulation: Operations, engineering, and management*. Burlington, MA: Elsevier.

4

THE SIMULATION OPERATIONS SPECIALIST AS INNOVATOR

S. Scott Atkinson
Summa Health, Akron, OH, USA

An understanding of the day-to-day challenges faced by the simulation operations specialist (SOS) is essential and warrants discussion. The challenges faced by the SOS include the constraints of budget, limited supplies, and general resources. In a simulation program, the thought processes required by the SOS to succeed are difficult to describe. Although experience may contribute greatly to the development of these thought processes, they also come from a mindset that is characteristic or part of the temperament of the individual. As career opportunities in simulation operations grow, many continuing and formal education programs are in development to help individuals build these characteristics in the classroom environment and with mental models.

SIMULATION OPERATIONS SPECIALISTS (SOS): WHERE DO THEY COME FROM?

Where do SOSs come from? This question challenges many simulation labs around the world. Good SOSs share similar characteristics. These individuals are:

- innovators,
- entrepreneurs,
- team players,

Healthcare Simulation: A Guide for Operations Specialists, First Edition.
Edited by Laura T. Gantt and H. Michael Young.
© 2016 John Wiley & Sons, Inc. Published 2016 by John Wiley & Sons, Inc.

- good communicators,
- creative and quick thinkers (resourceful),
- able to think from different perspectives.

Skill sets are certainly important for the SOS, but the *frame of mind*, or overall way of thinking—*mental processes* (MPs) are key factors in selecting an appropriate individual for a position on the operations team. The MPs of the SOS are demonstrated across simulation modalities and often link these individuals to their career choices. MPs emerge in individuals with backgrounds typically include characteristics listed in the bulleted list above. These skill sets are typically seen in those who come from the professional backgrounds in medicine, information technology (IT), audiovisual (AV), and performance arts, and persons who have a strong desire to do something new, to "make a difference."

For example, if asked to explain why Jim was hired into the position of SOS within a nursing simulation center, his supervisor would begin by saying that Jim was previously employed in instructional technology within a nursing school. Over time, the school recognized the need to have dedicated technology support for its clinical skills and simulation labs. The school has a wide array of technology-rich teaching tools, including human patient simulators and virtual reality software. Jim was hired to be the SOS for the nursing school because of his track record of providing timely help to the labs by troubleshooting complex networking platform issues related to simulators and video recording. In addition, Jim has shown a propensity for working with faculty and equipment vendors to modify manikins to meet specific learning objectives for students by using ballistic gelatin and individual molds that he creates. The school has expressed interest in working with Jim to patent some of his creations. Jim's expertise is sought within and from outside the school.

An analysis of the MPs necessary to supplement the skill sets of individuals like Jim shows that each of them possesses key characteristics which favor their becoming successful as an SOS. One identified *MP* in all of these individuals is that they are mental "mechanics." When the situation arises to fix a problem, it can be done quickly and with little error. These individuals feel a strong desire to be recognized for their contributions and this, in turn, drives their passion for success.

Operations specialist roles are often filled by instructional or information technology specialists, physicians, nurses, EMTs, paramedics, firefighters, allied health specialists, educators, biomedical engineers, and artists. The skill sets associated with such roles have been thought to best align with those required of the SOS. While few individuals will fulfill all expectations of a proposed job, an examination of individual traits, skills, and knowledge will help identify the best candidate.

Three main factors that will influence departmental leadership when hiring an SOS:

1. How many persons are in the existing simulation program? (faculty, staff, learners/participants)

2. Is the candidate teachable? In other words, can certain skills and knowledge be taught (transferred) to a new person on the team?
3. What salary range can be supported by the simulation program budget?

Each of these factors will be discussed in subsequent sections.

Hiring and Training the New SOS

The numbers of current members within a simulation center will greatly affect decisions about hiring a new operations specialist. Larger simulation centers will usually have staff that includes a director, a coordinator, manager(s), educator(s), clerical staff, fellows, adjuncts, and other ancillary staff. If this is the case, there is more time and latitude for having existing staff teach the new SOS whatever components are necessary. For example, if hiring an operations specialist with an information technology (IT) background …

- the physician can teach medical and clinical concepts and terminology,
- the educator can teach curriculum design and learning theories,
- the administrative assistant can teach office management and supply ordering, and
- the new operations specialist can attend ACLS, BLS, and similar classes to gain basic medical teamwork strategies.

While hiring highly qualified medical and clinical staff can certainly bolster a simulation programs level of expertise, the cost of doing so may not be necessary. As one can see, a decent size simulation staff does not necessarily require hiring an additional physician or nurse to fill the operations specialist role. Experts from other fields can augment an already diverse operations team. On the other hand, without the ability to hire additional full-time staff, a simulation program with only one full-time, dedicated staff member may be forced to learn, and then teach the technical aspects of running scenarios on their own. Although this is not ideal, it will fill the need for basic simulation scenarios, but probably not without help from the institution's instructional technology department (or helpdesk) and vendor support. Once the simulation center begins to grow and expand, however, the simulation program's best interest is to hire one or more qualified operations specialist(s) in order to ensure that day-to-day operations are maintained successfully.

Funding the Position for a New SOS

Creating success does not have to come with a capital budget! Many simulation centers face budget constraints. The dollars that support simulation education have decreased over time in many places. Although this greatly affects the operations of the simulation center, it does not change the reality that the one resource that will potentially save the simulation center the most money *is* the operations specialist.

Remember the *MPs* discussed earlier? Many managers tend to overlook the hidden talents possessed by the operations specialist. Once the decision is made to hire the operations specialist, this individual will ideally possess the keys to success that a simulation program needs. Simulation program leadership must determine how best to extract those latent talents for best utilization within the center.

HOW MIGHT THE SOS BE BEST UTILIZED?

The operations specialist has the budget control "tricks" already built into their MPs. The operations specialist should always have three questions in mind:

1. "What is the objective?"
2. "What are my resources?"
3. "Where can I save money?"

These are known as "ORM" or *objectives*, *resources*, and *money*. Before discussing "ORM," the hiring manager must make sure the SOS has the *MPs* to create the ORM. To accomplish this, the SOS should have a general understanding of curriculum development, as well as the teaching and debriefing processes. While this statement may seem controversial for some, it is important to understand the value of professional development, teamwork, honest feedback and maximum potential for the SOS, other simulation program staff, and educators. The discussion of the operations specialist's MPs is the foundation for the operations specialist to address the "ORM" questions. The SOS will be unable to understand the simulation program or simulation session objectives without shared knowledge from the team's planning because this awareness helps the SOS know where the team wants to be at the launch of the session.

The SOS can best understand objectives by being involved in the educational planning process. Once the SOS understands what the educator wants from the session, the operations specialist can suggest and begin to plan the optimal route of delivery. The planning committee can also better understand available resources because they now realize the kind of available equipment, as well as equipment purchases which must be made to meet planned objectives. For example, a scenario that requires auscultation of bowel sounds in a 2-year-old "patient" is not possible with a simulator that does not have bowel sounds. The role of the SOS is to identify those features that a simulator can and cannot demonstrate and to communicate this with the simulation team as a whole.

Finally, financial aspects are where the MPs of the SOS may show resourcefulness and creativity. An example may prove helpful here. Operations specialist John Smith just attended a meeting with the educators of the obstetrics and gynecology (OB-GYN) department. The group discussed its need for a simulator to demonstrate a live birth followed by a neonatal resuscitation of the newly delivered neonate. $60,000 has been allocated for this purchase. The educators stated that they are ready to purchase the mannequin as soon as next week and be able to perform this simulation scenario once a month. The educators do not foresee any other uses for the mannequins. At $60,000, the monthly cost of using this technology is at least $5000 plus the cost of supplies and miscellaneous expenses. The educators further indicate that they would like to keep the new birthing mannequin at a satellite hospital where the scenarios will be implemented. After additional discussion, John proposes to buy a low-fidelity birthing mannequin that costs $5000 plus a $1000 mannequin (neonate) to teach neonatal resuscitation. John states that there is no need to purchase the $60,000 simulator when the objective is only to perform a live birth and do neonatal resuscitation. He will also provide vital signs using free software from a tablet-based application to simulate the monitor. John used his *MPs* to demonstrate both innovation and an entrepreneurial spirit. John also used ORM to understand the educators' objectives, identified available resources, and saved a total of $54,000 for the school.

While John's resourcefulness is to be applauded, it is equally important to recognize that this same situation should have been handled differently if the circumstances were altered. For example, what if the OB-GYN educators were also planning on instructing midwifery students and identified additional learner objectives that necessitated a higher level of mannequin fidelity? What if the group also were aware that a new orientation curricula additional new hires would support weekly use of a birthing mannequin? In these cases, John would likely use ORM to evaluate the situation in a new light and recommend that the group proceed with purchase of the much more expensive, but more versatile, birthing mannequin.

THE SOS OF THE FUTURE

With an understanding of the operations specialist's MPs and "ORM" that supports it, where will an employer find the SOS of the future? The healthcare simulation field is still in the process of developing potentially successful educational and career paths for the SOS. The Society for Simulation in Healthcare (SSH) and its affiliates have developed a professional certification for the growing specialty of simulation operations: the *Certified Healthcare Simulation Operations Specialist* (CHSOS). Consequently, this new certification is beginning to highlight the likelihood that in the very near future, universities and colleges will launch accredited courses and degree programs to prepare the operations specialists for new professional horizons.

Although the development and successes of these programs are monumental landmarks in the operations specialists' potential career paths, a comparison of the SOS career path to other professions sheds light on the timeline. An in-depth look at the field of nursing's career development, where it started, and where it is today provides a worthwhile comparison to the SOS's career development.

The Evolution of Professional Nursing: 1855—Nightingale fund established for nurse training

- 1860—First nurses begin formal training
- 1919—First state registration for nursing

To date, the profession of nursing is 160 years old (LA History Archive, 2009).

The Evolution of Simulation (Rosen, 2008):

- 1960—First simulator was developed for anesthesia
- 1990—High-fidelity simulators hit the market
- 1990—Present medical simulation EXPLODES

Medical simulators have existed for 45 years.

This timeline provides an understanding of how quickly the SOS's opportunities for advancement are developing. Nursing has been around for 160 years to date, with state registration documenting an understanding of various nursing concepts and skills accomplished over the last 60 years. In comparison, simulation laboratories exploded in the early 1990s, presenting the need for the emergence of the SOS role. These careers are just now laying the foundation for the development of formal education for the SOS, which means that the SOS has had only 25 years to accomplish what other professions have taken twice as long to achieve.

CONCLUSION

Obtaining a greater knowledge of the SOS comes through the understanding of their individuality, background, hidden or latent talents, and mental thought processes. These individuals have an outstanding opportunity to gain additional knowledge through formal and informal educational resources that will contribute to earning greater respect and simulation program sustainability provided by the current and emerging simulation operations workforce. While many programs do not have a dedicated simulation workforce, one can observe that those who enjoy the multi-faceted presence of a knowledgeable and skilled operations specialist improve faculty buy-in and implementation of simulation best-practices and standards. While the role of a dedicated simulation educator is long overdue for ANY simulation program, it is equally true that what one professional lacks in technological skills and innovation is balanced by the hiring of a good SOS. The SOS should be one of the first two full-time roles created for a successful simulation program. The idea that hundreds of thousands of dollars, if not millions of dollars are spent on equipment and facilities while making staffing and training a lower priority is unfortunate, but is more common than one might think. However, as long as grants are written to finance the purchase of equipment and building facilities, but not the professionals needed to operate such a program, this practice is likely not to change any time soon.

REFERENCES

LA History Archive. (2009). *The western conservancy of nursing history timeline*. Retrieved June 24, 2015, from http://lahistoryarchive.org/resources/WCNH_Timeline/index.html

Rosen, K. R. (2008). The history of medical simulation. *Journal of Critical Care, 23*(2), 157–166.

5

THE SIMULATION OPERATIONS SPECIALIST AS ARTIST AND PRODUCER

EMILY SHAW

Mimic Technologies, Simugreat, SAGES, Baltimore, MD, USA

A simulation program depends on the creativity and innovation of its staff members, including the simulation operations specialist (SOS), for assisting in custom simulator development, painting "pathologies" on standardized patients, and replicating the sights and sounds of a clinical environment. This chapter will discuss how artistic endeavor can enhance the fidelity of scenarios through moulage, or design of key visual and audio, to enhance environmental emersion.

MOULAGE

The French word for casting or creating molds is "moulage." In the world of simulation, the term has become synonymous with the art of creating artificial bruises, injuries, lacerations, bone breaks, impaled objects, or any other trauma that may befall the human body and require medical treatment. Moulage demands a lot of creativity, understanding of color, and can range from pre-made silicone pieces of skin with an injury embedded to free-hand painted bruises directly to the skin of a standardized patient. Hollywood has mastered the theatrics of fake blood, realistic tissue from silicone or latex products, and staging environmental effect or props to recreate a traumatic incident, thanks to the horror films having the allure that they do with the public. There is even a sideshow at Universal Studios devoted to

Healthcare Simulation: A Guide for Operations Specialists, First Edition.
Edited by Laura T. Gantt and H. Michael Young.
© 2016 John Wiley & Sons, Inc. Published 2016 by John Wiley & Sons, Inc.

moulage called the "Horror Makeup Show" which is both gruesome and entertaining. Before Hollywood, realistic rendering of trauma, diseases, and anatomy reach back into the Renaissance period with wax sculptures like those found at the Museo La Specula in Florence, Italy. One company that found its roots in clinical simulation through moulage was Laerdal Medical; the company moved in the 1950s from being a popular doll manufacturer to designing realistic wound simulators for emergency medical training. A list of moulage resources is found in Appendix 5 of the book.

ENVIRONMENTAL REALISM

Research has indicated that increased realism in the simulation environment can improve learning and performance (Donoghue et al., 2010; Dunnington, 2015), especially when the clinical environment is an area such as a military battle field. The Bethesda, Maryland-based USUHS Simulation Center, boasts of a high-end environmental battlefield simulator called the wide area virtual environment (WAVE) team training simulator. The WAVE is an 8000-square-foot, multi-axis forum that uses stereoscopic images that fully surround the scenario participants. Team members work together on team training with real equipment immersed in sights and sounds of what is their "real world" on the battlefield. 3D artists worked to create the interactive virtual environment that projects 360° around the participants, including a landscape, civilians, and treacherous environmental props. Not every simulation center can afford or has the team to develop such an extensive environmental simulator for each scenario or course offered. However, there are many ways that the staff can work together to create key environmental sensory cues and props that make the experience of treating a specific patient in a space more similar to the space in which they work on a day-to-day basis. "Behind the Sim Curtain" (see Appendix 5), in addition to being an excellent resource for moulaging ideas, also has a listing of simulation props, including simulated smoke, emesis trays, and methods for recreating seizures on mannequins. Backdrops for certain clinical environments can be inexpensively recreated with wall panels to replicate the inside of an ambulance, and wall-sized posters can be purchased that represent hospital walls. However, most simulation centers opt for realistic wall mounts and hospital walls that are functional with bare essentials, like a fake headwall that has air flow, but not necessarily actual oxygen flowing.

Sounds in the healthcare environment can provide cues or distractions, both of which are important for the learner to become familiar with and navigate as they focus on the priorities of treating their patient. Aside from recording live hospital or clinical environment sounds, there are some that can be found online prerecorded, such as ER background noise and some may come from free online libraries. Websites for these can also be found in Appendix 5.

The voice of the patient can be essential to the realism of the scenario. Several tools to help with this are either the built-in laptop microphone to patient simulator or piping in a voice that emits from the around the head of the patient via a pillow speaker or Karaoke machine. Of course, the most realistic of interactions would be with a standardized patient who is well trained on the pathologies of the patient that they represent.

Other than simulating the sights and sounds of a real clinical environment, smells and tactile components of a patient interaction can provide important clues toward successful diagnosis and treatment. Laerdal (see Appendix 5 for website information) provides a recipe book for different bodily fluids; food products like black cherry jam or jello used to simulate blood clots can provide impressive believability.

IN-HOUSE VERSUS CONTRACTED SIMULATOR DEVELOPMENT

When funding is not readily accessible for big purchases, when a procedure does not already have a simulation solution, or when the disposables for an available simulator are not sustainable on the operating budget, the question arises: "Do we purchase from a vendor or design our own simulator?" To answer this question, the following factors must be considered:

- annual operating budget,
- existing staffing commitments and turn-over,
- reliability of information provided by your subject matter expert (SME),
- accessibility of supplies for simulator development, and
- sustainability of either a do-it-yourself (DIY) solution or vendor-provided solution with a general idea of forecasted consumable use.

Once the simulation program objectives are defined, determining the best solution, the decision must often be based on whether a vendor or DIY solutions fits within a program's budget. The SOS can assist by initiating side-by-side comparison of the two or more options. To proceed, the SOS would determine the initial simulator purchase price from a vendor, cost of the annual warranty encompassing major fixes, consumables for invasive procedures, and maintenance supplies for minor fixes. All of these products should be compared to the cost of producing a DIY simulator and include ongoing parts replacement. The ongoing cost is to maintain a simulator purchased from a vendor can be difficult to gauge, unless it is possible to predict, for example, exactly how many sticks a simulator can take before needing a replacement skin, vein, or fluid reservoir. Complete transparency from the vendor about how much each component costs to replace and what is covered under warranty versus out-of-pocket expenses is also needed. Another challenge is anticipating and including the depreciation of technology over time for a vendor-purchased simulator, a concept so well understood for mobile computers, yet poorly defined for simulators. When considering a DIY alternative, as opposed to purchasing an off-the-shelf simulator, the SOS should look at the production work-flow and availability of supplies for developing anything in-house. Working relationships between SOSs and SMEs can sprout some truly innovative simulator designs. To ensure the development of a high-quality simulator in-house, adopt an effective design process from the beginning and model behaviors after those of a typical product development team.

Good ideas can come from the most unpredictable of sources, so gathering all talent in one location and brainstorming sessions are critical at the beginning of a project so that all voices are heard in an unbiased way. Rules of engagement for an effective brainstorming session are as follows:

1. Embrace that "no idea is a bad idea" and all ideas are valid until proven irrelevant.
2. Know that assumptions and biases are a reality for every participant and should be dealt with openly through active listening.
3. Understand that hierarchy should not get in the way of great ideas.
4. SME and end user opinions should both be weighted equally.
5. Admission of ignorance early in the process is more constructive and will help prevent slow production through the delay of the inevitable.
6. Diversity in professional background and techniques adds to greater potential for meeting the broadest market and training needs.

Before any brainstorming can occur, the team should understand the problem that is to be solved with an in-house DIY simulator and have a working knowledge of what training solutions already exist versus what can be built. When proposing a solution based on the outcome of your brainstorming session, be sure to "say what you mean and mean what you say" in order to ensure that the development team can fully understand the goals set forth in your plan for simulator development. The SOS can also help this process by developing a skills matrix of the simulation center's employees to ensure sufficient staff and skills to complete the project. One online resource for creating a skills matrix can be found by doing an Internet search for "How to Create a Skills Matrix" for Dummies.

Simulator Design Commences

If the design team has decided to create a custom simulator instead of purchasing from a vendor, they will be embarking on a *creative process* which should begin with a well-conceived general concept. Once the brainstorming session is complete and there is a goal set for the team, every team member should be given the autonomy needed to begin the design of a simulator or contribute in their individual project role. Mastery in this skill of designing, casting, molding, and producing will come with time and by learning from those who have had success before. A fresh perspective and attention to solving the problem at hand as opposed to replicating what has already been created by others will serve the production team well.

Functionality and sustainability of a DIY simulator should be maintained throughout the design process and all the way through embedding the custom simulator into clinical curricula. As the old adage says, "form follows function," this holds true with simulators as it does with human anatomy. Once the desired behaviors of the simulator are known, research into potential building materials may begin. The SOS and other operations team members should trust instincts and senses when selecting supplies to work with. Experimentation with conventional materials may result in highly realistic tissues, such as the combination of pulled cotton and vegetable oil which creates a beautiful, webby material that cannot easily be dissected except with electrocautery.

BUILDING A FOUNDATION OF RESOURCES

The SOS should develop a network of professionals as a support system early on in this simulator building process as in other aspects of the role. A non-disclosure agreement (NDA) should be considered for the development team and partners to sign to prevent concerns about intellectual property. The importance of sharing lessons learned from inside or outside your own area cannot be underestimated. What patterns can be seen in previous product design attempts by others? What techniques have worked? What has failed in the past? Embrace error and ask why the error occurred instead of steering immediately in a new direction, since errors may be an indication that the user is meeting a challenge with a DIY simulator that is more global than the immediate problem.

Estimating Development Time

As the SOS considers the long-term sustainability of a simulator, the behaviors of the full spectrum of learners who will be using it must be taken into consideration. An estimate of an average number of procedural attempts until success is reached by each learner can help predict when components will need to be replaced. Based on this information, determining the on-going maintenance requirements to replace parts can be estimated, as can a typical cost for each one of the simulator's disposable parts over time. This allows for the capture of the hours worked to rebuild the disposable pieces, as well as the time it takes the SOS to repair the simulator. This decides how to budget for parts and labor costs for repairs.

If a vendor's comparable simulator is not available in the simulation center in order to observe a user's behaviors and to determine maintenance needs, then a survey of other simulation centers or Society for Simulation in Healthcare (SSH) members is recommended. The ease of use for the person doing the procedure and the SOS working with the simulator over time are critical to create value, positive experiences, best learning outcomes, and building customer loyalty; this can be just as important for the operations team as for potential vendors who may later buy the simulator design.

Determine a Pool of SMEs

When creating a custom simulator, SMEs are needed to assist in design to ensure that the correct anatomy is represented and that relevant procedures can be performed on it. Otherwise, the simulator designer will have to become proficient in these areas.

This is necessary before full emersion with the "story" (procedure and learning process) can be recreated. The story should be played out to gain knowledge of what the full course of events that the simulator will be used for; for example, in a surgical simulation, how does care progress from preparation and pre-operative care to wound care and on-going care. If it is possible to market a "curriculum roadmap" alongside the newly created simulator, the whole package will be that much more valuable to the user or potential buyer; this can translate into satisfaction, successful integration, and a higher asking price for the simulator if it is later sold.

When designing a simulator, consider the following roles: the learner (tangibility, fidelity, clarity of key concepts), the educator (curriculum, ease of use), the SOS (technical support, maintenance, sustainability), the simulation center administration (justification/return on investment—ROI), and the potential vendor (distribution, value, profit margins). These roles represent viewpoints that a vendor typically considers; they also translate well into metrics for deciding between purchasing a simulator or designing a comparable simulator in-house.

Public Resources for Simulation

The experienced SOS knows the necessity of compiling simulation resources and talking with connections about design, utilization, repair, and maintenance of simulators on the path to finding operational success with any solution that may be purchased or designed in-house. In fact, resources should be identified before starting any simulation program to get a clear picture of what it costs to keep it fully operational over time. Professional networks, simulation experts, associations, local connections, and online resources should all be explored for appropriate mentors and partners.

Simulation networks that are available to the public are LinkedIn groups, including Clinical Simulation Network, Center for Medical Simulation Network, Healthcare Simulation Connection, Medical Training and Simulation, Simulation123-International Simulation Community; HealthySimulation, which includes Medical Simulation News and Resources; Medical Simulation User Network (Laerdal); SimGHOSTS, SimPortal, Society for Simulation in Healthcare (SSH), and other vendor sites.

Simulation society conferences and local chapter meetings offer excellent venues to connect with fellow simulation colleagues. SSH hosts a meeting every year called the International Meeting for Simulation in Healthcare (IMSH). The American College of Surgeons (ACS) Accredited Educational Institution annual consortium meeting in Chicago is well worth going to for insights into the global simulation needs of a broad spectrum of surgical disciplines that rarely meet under one roof. The NextMed MMVR (Medicine Meets Virtual Reality) conference is for those developing interactive simulators that involve virtual reality (VR) or other technology. If medical graphics for a simulator project are needed, the Association of Medical Illustrators (AMI) hosts certified medical artists proficient in a range of 2D/3D animation, graphic design, web design, 3D printing, anatomical sculpture, mobile apps, micro-simulators, VR technologies, storyboards, and digital/traditional illustrations derived from a working knowledge of anatomy.

Design Resources Close to Home

Helpful services for simulator development offered by local businesses may be useful for consultation, support, or outsourcing, including 3D printing and scanning companies, anatomy departments, local freelance medical illustrators, anaplastologists with knowledge in anatomical sculpting and silicone materials, simulator vendors, experienced simulation center operations and technology experts, and healthcare subject matter experts.

Local 3D printing companies can often respond more quickly to requests while meeting quality expectations and production timelines. Nearby engineering departments, art schools, or other simulation centers may have 3D printers available. If CT or MRI data sets of the anatomy can be obtained for a DIY simulator, local 3D scanning and printing services can be of great value and may significantly speed up the development process.

To obtain medical imaging data, a relationship must be developed with local anatomy departments for surface scanning of specimens or radiology departments for access to CT and MRI data sets with patient identifiers removed. Permission from these departments to share information may be prohibited by their institutional policies. Establishing a formal partnership with a hospital to develop simulators jointly may provide access to required anatomical data. Local medical illustrators may be helpful in this process, as they often settle near the medical schools where they trained and have relationships with the anatomy department or radiology that could be of benefit. There is a directory of medical illustrators on the AMI website (ami. org). Anaplastology, the art of restoring a malformed or absent part of the human body through artificial means, is often taught in conjunction with medical illustration programs. Anaplastologists also have strong connections to hospitals since they work with surgeons, radiologists, and use CT and MRI data to generate 3D models of patient's faces and limbs in order to design prosthetics. They also have detailed knowledge of silicone and mold-making techniques in order to fabricate prostheses that could also be helpful with simulator development.

HYBRID SOLUTIONS FOR SIMULATOR DEVELOPMENT

Hybrid solutions are available for outsourcing of parts or all of the development of a simulator. Such companies will work to generate digital 3D models and tangible prototypes of a concept for a DIY simulator. A production fee must be paid when working with such companies. How protection of intellectual property and generation of a patent would transpire in this scenario is not straightforward and should be investigated at the beginning of a working relationship.

Simulator Fabrication

When it is time to begin the fabrication of a DIY simulator, the concept must be outlined to ensure a thorough understanding of the product. With concept in hand, research into the existing market can be completed to determine if there is competition. If the product is deemed viable, assistance in drawing up your prototype can be accomplished by a freelance artist, medical illustrator, 3D modeler, or an expert with AutoCad. The simulator can then be modeled via 3D printing from CT/ MRI datasets, sculpted with oil-based clay for later mold making, or assembled with purchased components. This is an area where learning from other industries will be helpful, such as Hollywood special effects companies, online sculpting tutorials/ videos, calling up your local anaplastologist to ask for advice on manipulating silicone products and mold making.

TESTING YOUR DIY SIMULATOR

After the functionality of the prototype is determined, it can be fine-tuned to meet training needs. A focus group of SMEs who have signed an NDA to beta test the product with the goal of trying to "push it to the limit" to see what deficiencies may still exist, how much wear and tear it can handle, and how effective of a training tool it really is. Data points and feedback should be from the members of your beta testing team.

PROTECTING INTELLECTUAL PROPERTY

Patents should be filed by members of the simulator design team early in the process, especially if investors are sought for later stages in development. The US Patent Office's website provides step-by-step instructions on patents.

During the development of a custom simulator, each person's contribution should be logged for inclusion in patent submission and to give credit where credit is due when the product comes to fruition. Each contributor should be appropriately recognized for their part in the project and be able to promote their accomplishments in the professional domain. No one person should be allowed to overshadow the work of the team members who contributed ideas to the overall product.

FUNDING FUTURE DEVELOPMENT

After obtaining a patent, financial backing for the newly created simulator may be requested either internally through an employer or through a partnership with outside investors. The target audience will want to know what the maintenance, ROI, forecasting on disposables, and sustainability of the simulator may be, which will be challenging to provide prior to any initial utilization of the product. As much data as can be generated by vetting the simulator within an existing simulation center and other beta testing sites will be essential. Beta testing sites should also be required to sign an NDA to protect intellectual property, but are usually quite easy to find considering that their training centers will have access to a new simulator, without having to purchase it, in exchange for data. For simulator operational forecasting, determine the frequency that replacement parts are being built or ordered, and how many man hours it takes to build replacement parts as well as repair of non-disposable components. With this information, the SOS and other team members can determine whether it is possible to be self-sustaining with maintaining and building simulator disposables, or if a partnership with a vendor is required to produce disposables in order to sustain active use of the simulator.

When looking for a vendor to partner with, consider the company's history with partnerships, breadth of product offerings, and, if their target audience is in alignment with the newly designed simulator, as well as potential benefits being sought in the partnership. A partnership could span anywhere from handing over a patent to the vendor for the purpose of having fabrication taken over to partnering with a company that will help move idea for a simulator to a complete product for a fee or partial ownership. Partnership with a well-respected company that makes simulators can have many advantages; it can free up time to work on other ideas and may provide additional resources that would otherwise be expensive to pay for, such as product developers, legal services, product managers to help with market forecasting, relations and marketing resources, and high-end fabrication facilities. If the simulation operations team does not have the skills required to complete development of a prototype, partnering with a company that may not have a broad selection of simulators, but is small and dynamic with an excellent product development team may be beneficial.

CONCLUSION

In conclusion, thriving creativity of the SOS and other simulation center staff members can lead to successful outcomes with custom simulator development, more realistic disease presentation in scenarios through skilled moulaging, and the creation of convincing sights and sounds of environments within which patients are typically cared for. With the resources provided in this chapter, important connections can be made to enhance the creative capability of the team by complimenting existing in-house talent with external associations, online groups, companies, and vendors to enhance the experience of learners in an evolving simulation center.

REFERENCES

Donoghue, A. J., Durbin, D. R., Nadel, F. M., Stryjewski, G. R., Kost, S. I., & Nadkarni, V. M. (2010). Perception of realism during mock resuscitations by pediatric housestaff: The impact of simulated physical features. *Simulation in Healthcare, 5*(1), 16–20.

Dunnington, R. M. (2015). The centricity of presence in scenario-based high fidelity human patient simulation: A model. *Nursing Science Quarterly, 28,* 64–73.

6

MEDICAL AND CLINICAL TERMINOLOGY FOR THE SIMULATION OPERATIONS SPECIALIST

MORGAN SCHERWITZ[1], CHERYL HUNTER[2], LINDSEY SCOTT[3], AND LAURA T. GANTT[4]

[1] *Hendrick Hospital, Abilene, TX, USA*
[2] *Tarleton State University, Stephensville, TX, USA*
[3] *Consultant, Austin, TX, USA*
[4] *East Carolina University College of Nursing, Greenville, NC, USA*

All professions develop their own language, jargon, and idioms that only those in the profession can understand. Often this language is used without considering whether or not it is understood by others in the conversation, which can lead to a great deal of confusion. This is especially problematic if understanding the language is necessary for the completion of a task or direction. In essence, it is like being in a foreign country and trying to understand a native's directions to the nearest hotel. The language of medicine can be just as impenetrable as French or Russian is to English-only speaking Americans. As is the case with foreign languages, regional and cultural influences may make an understanding of medical language that much more challenging.

As with any language, learning its more common terms is a good place to start on the road to medical language competency. Just as important to gaining comprehension and mastery is understanding the root of the words and the context in which they

Healthcare Simulation: A Guide for Operations Specialists, First Edition.
Edited by Laura T. Gantt and H. Michael Young.
© 2016 John Wiley & Sons, Inc. Published 2016 by John Wiley & Sons, Inc.

are most often used. Integrating medical language into the healthcare simulation education context is especially challenging. Essentially, simulation requires that two or more people understand one another that likely may come from different professional backgrounds. In this particular case, the concern is that the simulation operations specialist (SOS) and healthcare professionals may not be communicating in a common language, which may detract from establishing quality learning experiences.

The purpose of this chapter is to review body systems and the associated terms that the SOS might encounter. In order to participate in the design of instructional experiences with human patient simulators, the SOS must be able to realistically adjust human physiologic and pathophysiologic parameters within the mannequin and its software.

THE BRAIN AND CENTRAL NERVOUS SYSTEM

Root word	*neur*—nerve (Chabner, 2015)

The Central Nervous System and Altered Mental Status

The central nervous system (CNS) pertains to the brain, cerebrospinal fluid, cerebellum, and brain stem. Any issues within the CNS may lead to *altered mental status* or AMS. Common causes of AMS may include head trauma, insufficient blood flow caused by things such as stroke or low blood pressure, low blood sugar, infection, and fever. A variety of methods can be employed in the assessment of a patient's mental status. Healthcare professionals will often start checking mental status to determine a patient's ease of arousal or wakefulness. Clients with AMS are usually difficult to wake up and may need to have a painful stimulus applied to get a response. Orientation to person, place, time, and situation are generally the next step of assessing mental status. Individuals that have AMS may have speech issues as evidenced by slurring of words or difficulty answering questions. When answering questions, the client may be confused and may provide inappropriate responses.

Peripheral Nervous System

Neuropathy refers to a decrease in sensation as a result of nerve impairment, and can also be responsible for chronic pain. This can be caused by trauma, lack of blood flow to capillaries as in the case of uncontrolled diabetes, and other nervous system diseases. Sensation includes the ability to feel pain, heat and cold, fine touch and deep pressure. Any or all of these sensations may be affected in a client who suffers from neuropathy regardless of its cause.

Cerebrovascular Accident (CVA)   A CVA is more commonly known as a *stroke*. Strokes can be either caused by a clot or bleeding from a blood vessel that supplies the brain tissue with oxygen. The lack of oxygen causes cellular death and injury, which leads to impaired or absent function from the damaged area. Signs and symptoms of stroke include the following:

- a change in mental status,
- impaired speech or movement (such as paralysis on only one side of the body (hemiplegia)), and
- visual changes.

The gold standard for assessing the severity of stroke is the National Institute of Health Stroke Scale that can be viewed at http://www.ninds.nih.gov/doctors/nih_stroke_scale.pdf (National Institute of Health [NIH], 2003).

Transient Ischemic Attacks (TIAs)   A TIA is often referred to as a *mini-stroke*. This occurs when there is brief interruption in the blood flow to an area of the brain as a result of clots impeding blood flow. A patient experiencing a TIA will show all the signs of a stroke, but blood flow is spontaneously regained after a short time. This occurs when the clot is destroyed by chemicals that are naturally produced by the body. These lysing chemicals cause dissolution and are created by the body to get rid of clots.

Example of How Brain and CNS Problems Can be Simulated

An educator approaches the SOS with student learning objectives related to patients with stroke-like symptoms. The SOS explains that even the higher fidelity, more sophisticated simulation mannequin is not able to mimic hemiplegia, unless he/she is "conscious" and asked to respond to certain types of questions like "can you squeeze my hands?" However, the SOS notes that following stroke or neurologic symptoms *can* be simulated (see accompanying Fig. 6.1):

- Eyes half-closed or completely closed;
- Changes to pupillary reaction on eye exam;
- Garbled speech or loss of ability to use language;
- Unresponsiveness or other changes to mental status:
- Increased or decreased blood pressure.

The educator and SOS may also choose to use a standardized patient (simulated patient, SP) who develops increased intracranial pressure. Over the course of the scenario, the patient becomes progressively less able to respond to questions and stimuli, has increasing blood pressure, and then develops an extremely dilated pupil in one eye. In the case of using an SP, vitals and other symptoms can be emulated using a virtual patient monitor or specialized programmable instruments.

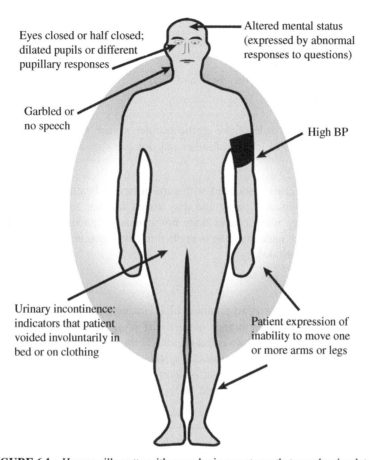

FIGURE 6.1 Human silhouette with neurologic symptoms that may be simulated.

The Cardiovascular System

This cardiovascular system is the body system that is composed of the heart and blood vessels that deliver blood to the body (Brooks & Brooks, 2014).

Root words	*cardio*—relating to the heart (Chabner, 2015)

Context

Patients experiencing cardiovascular, or problems with the heart and blood vessel, often complain of a variety of symptoms, including:

- shortness of breath,
- chest pain,
- sweating,
- nausea,

- coughing,
- upper back pain,
- extremity swelling,
- a strange "fluttering" in the chest, and
- anxiety.

Because of the central role of the cardiovascular system in all bodily functions, cardiac problems tend to impact all other physiologic systems, sometimes making diagnosis difficult.

Common Terms   Terms associated with cardiovascular health problems are used in mainstream conversation today and may sound familiar to the general public. However, familiarity with a term does not equate to understanding, which is important to how that understanding is applied in any situation that includes cardiac physiology or pathophysiology.

Pulse

The pulse is a result of the heart pumping blood through the body via vessels called *arteries*. These arteries expand and contract with blood at each pump of the heart, which can be felt or *palpated* at several regions of the body (see Table 6.1).

The pulse is evidence of cardiovascular system function and counting the pulse as it is palpated provides the heart rate. A heart rate is reported as beats per minute (bpm) and is normally between 60 and 100 bpm in adults. There are instances when the heart rate is too fast or too slow.

Root	*cardio*—relating to the heart
	brady—slow
	tachy—fast (Chabner, 2015)

Bradycardia is the term used for a heart rate *less than* 60 bpm; it can have several causes. Many athletes have resting heart rates less than 60 bpm with no ill effects

TABLE 6.1   Common Pulse Sites[a]

Site	Location
Carotid	Left and right side of the neck
Apical	Left chest just below the nipple (May be difficult to feel at this site but can be heard with a stethoscope)
Brachial	Inside bend of the elbow
Radial	At the right and left wrist below the thumb
Femoral	Right and left groin
Popliteal	Behind right and left knee
Posterior tibial	Inner side of right and left ankle
Dorsalis pedis	Top of right and left foot

[a]From Potter et al. (2012).

due to good cardiac conditioning. However, bradycardia can also be evidence of serious health issues such as drug overdose (or interaction), electrolyte imbalance, or hypothermia. *Tachycardia* refers to a heart rate *greater than* 100 bpm. As with bradycardia, there are several potential reasons for tachycardia. Exercise causes increased heart rate as does fever, pain, some forms of drug overdose or interaction, emotional state, electrolyte imbalances, and asthma (Huether & McCance, 2012; Potter, Perry, Stockert, & Hall, 2012).

Blood Pressure

Blood pressure is the result of the force of the heart pushing blood through the cardiovascular system's arteries. As the heart pumps or contracts, pressure in the arteries *increases* and between contractions, *decreases*. At the height of the contraction the pressure is the greatest and represents the *systolic pressure*. The heart rests at the end of each contraction resulting in less pressure and represents the *diastolic pressure*. Blood pressure is represented by a pair of numbers with the systolic on the top and the diastolic on the bottom. A normal blood pressure for an adult is 120/80. It is common for blood pressure results to be above or below normal (Potter et al., 2012).

Root	*tension*—pressure
	hyper—above, excessive
	hypo—below, deficient (Chabner, 2015)

A patient is considered *hypertensive* when their blood pressure is greater than 140/90. Patients with hypertension may not experience any side effects and may not know they have hypertension; those who do may complain of headache and blurred vision. There are multiple risk factors for hypertension, including:

- family history,
- gender,
- smoking,
- drinking,
- diabetes,
- race (African Americans have a higher incidence), and
- a diet high in salt.

Hypotension occurs when the systolic blood pressure (upper number in the blood pressure ration) is less than 90. Although some adults are normally hypotensive, it is not a normal finding. Hypotension causes patients to feel dizzy, especially when changing positions from sitting to standing. Patients with significant hypotension are confused, clammy, pale in appearance and may also have decreased urine output. These symptoms are life threatening and need immediate attention by a healthcare provider. Hypotension can be a result of:

- drug overdose or interaction,
- dehydration,

- physical exhaustion,
- starvation,
- illness,
- prolonged immobility, and
- pregnancy (Huether & McCance, 2012; Potter et al., 2012).

Heart Sounds

Blood flows into and out of the heart through a system of veins and arteries. This flow is regulated by the opening and closing of four valves that are located at the entrance and exit of each of the fours chambers of the heart. The flow of the blood and action of the valves as the heart contracts can be heard as "lub dub" when listening to the heart using a stethoscope. Occasionally, due to disease or genetics, the valves fail to open or close properly. This produces additional sounds called *murmurs* or *gallops*. Murmurs are heard as swishing or blowing sounds. Gallops are heard as an extra sound in the "lub dub" cycle and produce a rhythm and tone similar to the words "Kentucky" or "Tennessee" when spoken (Huether & McCance, 2012; Potter et al., 2012).

Cardiac Rhythms

The rhythmic beating of the heart is a result of electrical impulses that originate within the heart and are transmitted along electrical pathways to *firing nodes* that initiate the contraction of the heart muscle. Electrodes placed strategically on the chest capture the electrical activity in the heart and transmit the signal to the electro-cardiograph that results in an electrical picture of the heart, referred to as an electro-cardiogram (ECG), EKG, or a 12-lead. An ECG or EKG depicts the heart's electrical activity on a graph as lines and waves. A single beat of the heart is seen as a line with a complex of waves of varying elevations. Each part of the "QRS" complex is identified by a letter and represents a specific moment in time within the conduction (cardiac rhythm) process (Huether & McCance, 2012; Potter et al., 2012). See EKG diagram below.

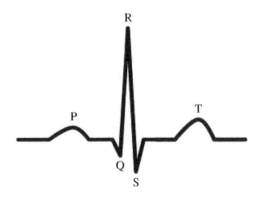

Diagram of Electrocardiogram (ECG) The P wave represents electrical activity in the top chambers (atria) of the heart. The QRS complex depicts electrical activity in the bottom chambers (ventricles) of the heart. The T wave represents the ventricles returning to rest after a contraction (Huether & McCance, 2012; Potter et al., 2012).

A disruption in the heart's electrical system causes a disruption in its rhythm. This disruption or irregularity is known as dysrhythmia (Huether & McCance, 2012; Potter et al., 2012). Another word for a *dysrhythmia* is an *arrhythmia*.

Root	*rhythmia*—rhythm
	dys—abnormal, painful (Chabner, 2015)

Dysrhythmias occur for a variety of reasons. Although some dysrhythmias are common and cause few or no ill effects, other dysthymias are life threatening if left untreated. Dysrhythmias appear in the ECG as alterations in the QRS wave complex and are clues to the underlying disease process. See Table 6.2.

Example of How Cardiovascular Problems Can be Simulated

The medical director of the hospital's Emergency Medical Services (EMS) approaches the SOS to assist in developing a simulation session for paramedics. The learning objectives involve review and management of less common cardiac dysrhythmias, such as supraventricular tachycardia (SVT) and pulseless electrical activity (PEA). The SOS discusses the availability of pre-programmed (programmed) scenarios for certain cardiac conditions and explains that high-fidelity simulators usually have a menu of normal and abnormal heart rhythms that can be displayed on a monitor. The simulator can also mimic heart sounds for auscultation and has palpable pulses in several key areas of the simulator's physiology, all of which may decrease or become absent to accommodate various clinical situations. The simulator also has the ability to measure volume and monitor specific medication during administration. The EMS medical director and the SOS choose a scenario in which the patient has SVT that deteriorates to PEA. The patient simulator will receive cardiac and BP monitoring, possibly cardioversion and endotracheal intubation, several types of medications, and intravenous (IV) fluids (see accompanying Fig. 6.2).

Capillary Refill

Capillary refill or *cap refill* refers to the ability of the capillaries to rebound after pressure is placed on a superficial area of the skin. When medical professionals are assessing this, they will often push on the nail bed briefly so that it becomes pale, then release the pressure and count how long it takes the area to return to its original state. In a healthy individual, the capillaries should refill in 3 seconds or less. If there

TABLE 6.2   Heart Rhythms

Rhythm	Causes	Considerations
Normal sinus rhythm	Healthy normal state	None
ST elevation myocardial infarction (STEMI)	Heart disease, lack of oxygen, or lack of blood supply to the heart	STEMI is life threatening if left untreated. It is commonly referred to as an MI or heart attack
Atrial flutter (AF)	Heart disease, heart attack, or drug toxicity	AF is not usually life threatening but is often treated to prevent deterioration into a more serious dysrhythmia
Atrial fibrillation (A-fib)	Heart disease, heart attack, or excessive alcohol or caffeine use	A-fib is not usually life threatening unless left untreated, and the patient becomes unstable
Supraventricular tachycardia (SVT)	Stimulants such as caffeine, nicotine, or amphetamines	SVT is not usually life threatening unless left untreated and the patient becomes unstable
Torsades de pointes	Heart disease, heart attack, or drugs	Torsades is a life-threatening condition that must be treated
Ventricular tachycardia (V-tach)	Heart attack, advanced heart disease, electrical shock, drugs, or severe lack of blood flow to the heart	V-tach is a life-threatening condition that must be treated
Ventricular fibrillation (V-fib)	Severe heart disease, electrical shock, or drug overdose	V-fib is a life-threatening condition and must be treated
Asystole	Untreated V-tach or V-fib, heart attack, advance heart disease, or electrical shock	Asystole is fatal and must be treated immediately
Pulseless electrical activity (PEA)	Severe blood loss, lack of oxygen, or heart muscle damage	PEA is fatal and must be treated immediately

Adapted from Atwood, Stanton, and Storey-Davenport (2013). © 2013 by James and Bartlett Learning.

is some circulatory problem, there may be a delay in capillary refill. The major causes of decreased capillary refill time are:

- trauma,
- damage or blockage to blood vessels leading to part of the body, and
- hypovolemia (low blood volume), or
- anemia (low hemoglobin).

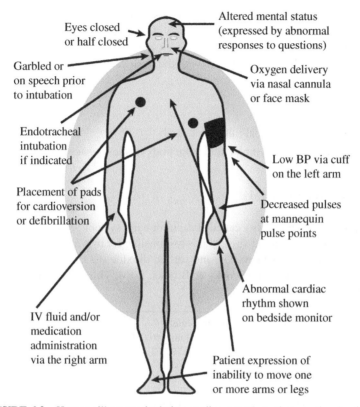

Eyes closed or half closed

Altered mental status (expressed by abnormal responses to questions)

Garbled or on speech prior to intubation

Oxygen delivery via nasal cannula or face mask

Endotracheal intubation if indicated

Low BP via cuff on the left arm

Placement of pads for cardioversion or defibrillation

Decreased pulses at mannequin pulse points

IV fluid and/or medication administration via the right arm

Abnormal cardiac rhythm shown on bedside monitor

Patient expression of inability to move one or more arms or legs

FIGURE 6.2   Human silhouette depicting cardiac symptoms that may be simulated.

DEEP VEIN THROMBOSIS (DVT)

Root word	*thromb*—clot (Chabner, 2015)

Deep vein thrombosis is seen when a clot forms in the deep veins most commonly in the lower legs and occasionally in the upper arms. A thrombus is a clot that forms on the side of a vessel as a result of stagnant blood, increased clotting factors in the blood, or injury to the vessel. The most common causes for DVTs are immobility, smoking, varicose veins, family history, clotting disorders, and age.

EDEMA

Root word	*edema*—swelling

Edema is a general term for swelling. Swelling can be acute, meaning localized or generalized, meaning found throughout the body. Edema is graded from 0, meaning none up to four in degrees of severity. The assessment of swelling is done through pushing on the affected area and noting how deep it appears. When the tissue does not rebound after the assessment, leaving an indentation, this is known as *pitting edema*. Edema can have many causes with the most common being such as:

- heart failure,
- trauma,
- electrolyte or nutritional imbalance, and
- kidney disease or a lymph (fluid from body tissues) system dysfunction.

RESPIRATORY SYSTEM

The respiratory system, also called the pulmonary system, consists of the lungs, airway or trachea, and blood vessels; it is responsible for moving air in and out of the lungs and exchanging oxygen (O_2) and carbon dioxide (CO_2) between the environment and the blood stream (Brooks & Brooks, 2014; Huether & McCance, 2012; Potter et al., 2012).

Root	*pulmon*—lung
	ary—pertaining to (Chabner, 2015)

Context

Patients who suffer from respiratory system issues experience many of the same symptoms as patients with heart problems, but for different reasons. This is not surprising, as the heart and lungs work together to supply the body with oxygen and blood. Unfortunately, this also means that each is greatly influenced by the health and effectiveness of the other. Respiratory problems commonly present as shortness of breath, fatigue, confusion, anxiety, cough, and decreased appetite.

Common Terms

While breathing is something everyone does with very little thought, in actuality, breathing is a complex process that occurs at the cellular level. Although many of the terms used to discuss the respiratory process are familiar, they often have different implications and meanings to those in healthcare. Understanding the technical meaning of these terms is essential in planning and implementing a simulation scenario that involves respiratory problems.

Respirations

Respiration refers to the process of inhaling and exhaling air. A normal respiratory rate differs according to age. Infants breathe fairly fast at a rate of 35–40 breaths per minute, while a normal respiratory rate for an adult is 12–20 breaths per minute.

There are instances when respirations are faster or slower than normal or are irregular or difficult (Huether & McCance, 2012; Potter et al., 2012).

Root	*pnea*—breathing
	brady—slow
	tachy—fast
	a—absence of, without
	dys—abnormal, painful (Chabner, 2015)

Dyspnea refers to any change from normal respiration and is more a description of the quality of the respirations than of breath regularity or rate. Patients presenting with dyspnea appear to be "working" to breathe or have "labored" breathing. This work of breathing is evidenced by flared nostrils, the retraction or pulling back of the muscles between the ribs with each breath, and using all the upper body to get air into the lungs. Dyspnea can be due to various factors including pain, anxiety, disease, or trauma (Huether & McCance, 2012; Potter et al., 2012).

Pulmonary Embolism

A pulmonary embolism (PE) occurs when blood clots build up in the vessels of the lungs. The most common cause of a PE is *deep vein thrombosis* (DVT). When such clots move from the legs, they travel up toward the heart and become stuck in the vessels of the lungs. A thrombus is called an embolus if it dislodges and travels to a new location.

Example of How Respiratory Problems Can be Simulated

A pulmonologist (pulmonary physician) contacts the SOS about teaching medical students how to recognize and manage a patient presenting with pulmonary embolus. The pulmonologist and SOS develop a scenario in which a patient with a DVT begins to manifest symptoms of a PE. The SOS recommends that there be a wound-like area on the calf of the mannequin's leg to simulate the DVT. The changes in mental status common to patients with PE can be simulated initially with increased anxiety and then with decreased responsiveness to questions and closed eyes. The mannequin's bedside monitor can show hypotension, decreased oxygen saturation, increased heart rate, and rapid respiratory rate. The simulator program allows for changes in breath sounds, including the lung crackles associated with PE.

GASTROINTESTINAL SYSTEM

The *gastrointestinal* (GI) system encompasses the path that nutrients take when they enter the body via the mouth as they pass through digestion in the stomach, small and large intestines and then exit the body via the rectum. This system is one that may exhibit symptoms even if not directly affected. For instance, a patient with a myocardial infarction (heart attack) may display nausea even though the direct injury is occurring to the heart and not the gastrointestinal system. Bowel sounds can be heard when a stethoscope is placed in the abdomen. Typically, a practitioner will listen to four quadrants of the abdomen. Visualize the abdomen and draw a line vertically across the umbilicus (belly button) and horizontally through the umbilicus, thus dividing the abdomen into four quadrants. These are the areas listened to by a practitioner for abdominal sounds.

Normoactive or normal bowel sounds are those heard in a healthy person. Normoactive sounds occur 5–35 times a minute and are created by air and fluids moving though the intestines (Potter et al., 2012). These sounds occur as a soft gurgling or bubbling noise and are a sign of a normal bowel function in a healthy patient.

Slower than normal sounds are described as *hypoactive* (hypo meaning slow) and may be caused by anesthesia after surgery. *Hypoactive* bowel sounds should be monitored as they may develop into *absent* bowel sounds. If there are no sounds present in the abdomen, then these are considered absent bowel sounds, which indicates lack of *peristalses* or *intestinal movement* typically caused by bowel obstruction (blockage of bowel) or *paralytic ileus* (temporary non-movement of the abdominal wall) (Potter et al., 2012).

Bowel sounds that occur more frequently than normoactive sounds are considered *hyperactive*. These are usually caused by GI upset or inflammation. Sounds that progress into an even more hyperactive state are called *borborygmi*. These are loud and "growling" in nature and can occur almost constantly when listening to the abdomen. Borborygmi are caused by diarrhea and ingestion of laxatives (Potter et al., 2012).

Conditions of the Gastrointestinal System

Nausea is the upset stomach feeling (queasy) that typically precedes vomiting. However, not every instance of nausea results in vomiting. Nausea can be the result of a virus, inflammation of the stomach lining due to consumption of food that was not cooked properly, or administration of an oral medication which causes an inflammatory response in the stomach.

Vomiting or *emesis* is the body's process of removing any substance from the stomach via the mouth. Like nausea, vomiting may occur due to infection from a virus or bacteria that causes inflammation in the stomach with subsequent rapid *peristalsis*. Vomiting can also be the result of increased stomach acid that the body cannot pass through the GI system quickly enough and must expel.

Both *nausea* and *vomiting* can be a sign of an injury that is not directly related to the GI system. For instance, a concussion, which is a bruising in the brain tissue, can cause nausea and vomiting even though there is nothing directly wrong with the GI system.

Root word	*emesis*—expelling matter from the stomach through the mouth
	hyper—excessive

Hyperemesis is an excessive amount of vomiting. For instance, if a person is unable to keep anything in their stomach due to vomiting, has uncontrolled nausea, and is losing sleep due to their inability to cease vomiting, they have entered a state of hyperemesis. An instance where this might occur is in *hyperemesis gravidarum* (excessive vomiting during pregnancy), which is vomiting and nausea beyond that which is typical with morning sickness. Pregnant women may be hospitalized due to risk of dehydration and secondary complications when vomiting becomes excessive.

Constipation

Bowel movements which occur infrequently, or less often than every 3 days, and are hard and require straining to pass are a sign of *constipation* (Potter et al., 2012). Constipation occurs quite frequently after surgery due to the administration of anesthesia, which causes the movement of the intestines to slow. Additionally, surgery usually causes painful movement, which leads to a patient avoiding the act of moving or walking. Walking and movement stimulate the intestines to move and pass stool, and if movement is limited, then stool will not pass as frequently. Narcotic pain medications also have a slowing effect on the intestines.

BOWEL OBSTRUCTION

A condition in which feces are unable to pass or progress in its normal flow down the intestines is called a *bowel obstruction*. Bowel obstructions may be caused by severe constipation or an *impaction* (collection of hard feces wedged in the rectum). The severity of a bowel obstruction can necessitate a range from treatments such as administration of laxatives and enemas to surgical removal.

Ostomy

In some conditions, such as cancer, stool passage through normal routes is no longer possible. When this occurs, a temporary or permanent opening is established that brings the intestines to the abdominal wall and creates an opening for feces to drain, the location of an ostomy in relation to where it occurs in the body. In this case, the location in the intestines will dictate the name. For instance, a surgical opening in the colon is a *colostomy*.

Diarrhea

Frequently occurring, liquid stools are *diarrhea*. Cramping and a feeling of an upset stomach may occur in conjunction with diarrhea. Diarrhea occurs when the gastrointestinal system is trying to rid itself of something harmful. For instance, the ingestion of contaminated food products can cause diarrhea because the body is attempting to expel this food as quickly as possible.

Nasogastric Tube

A *nasogastric tube* may be inserted in an attempt to drain or decrease pressure in the stomach. The flexible tube may be inserted through the nose, down the esophagus, and into the stomach. The tube can be left open to drain, clamped off, or suction may be applied to the tube. Medications and nutrients can also be administered via this tube. The tube is taped to the nose and special care must be taken to ensure it is located in the stomach and not the lungs prior to using this tube. The main way to check it is in the correct place is by X-ray.

PEG Tube

A *PEG tube* is a tube that is inserted directly into the stomach from the outside of the body and allows administration of nutrients, fluids, and medications. This tube allows nutrients to bypass the mouth and esophagus and is used at times with a patient who does not have the strength or desire to eat, such as those in hospice care (end of life care).

GENITOURINARY SYSTEM

The *genitourinary* system encompasses the organs which assist in creating and expelling fluid (urine) from the body and the genital organs. *Urine* is a waste product, which contains excess fluid, electrolytes, and other liquefied substances no longer needed by the body. Urine is pulled from the bloodstream by the kidneys and then carried to the bladder via the *ureters* (small tube that connects the kidney to the bladder). The *urethra* is the tube that carries urine from the bladder to the outside of the body. Typically, urine is clear, yellow to amber in color, has an acidic pH, and is not *malodorous* (unpleasant odor).

Bloody Urine

Severe bladder infections can cause irritation and bleeding of the bladder which seeps into the urine. Blood tinged urine is often red or pink in appearance. Certain medications such as blood thinners can cause bleeding into the urine. Also, foods such as beets can cause a pink/red tinge to the urine. The severity of the problem is indicated by the urine's depth of the color.

Urinary Tract Infection (UTI)

A *urinary tract infection* is often known as a *bladder infection*. Although often times it is the bladder that is infected, at times, other organs of the urinary tract may be infected as well, such as the kidneys, ureters, or urethra. Most UTIs occur in women. A UTI may also start as an infection of the urethra and progress upwards toward the bladder or kidneys.

Foley Catheter

A *Foley catheter* is a flexible tube that is inserted into the urethra and extends to the bladder. It facilitates the release of urine from the body. A Foley catheter is often placed during surgery to empty a patient's bladder while they are under anesthesia. It typically remains in place until the patient is able to move well enough to walk to the bathroom. Foley catheter insertion is a sterile procedure and great care must be maintained in not contaminating the tube that goes into the bladder. Should the tube be contaminated, a UTI will ensue.

MUSCULOSKELETAL SYSTEM

The *musculoskeletal* system includes anything pertaining to the system that gives the body its structure including bones, muscles, ligaments, and tendons.

Large Deformities

When a medical professional is assessing a patient, they first observe through inspection. A cursory inspection should reveal any large deformities to the musculo-skeletal system. Deformities may include any obvious changes in symmetry, swelling in a confined area, or a limb positioned inappropriately. One such deformity that is quite obvious includes a *femoral head fracture*. This is when the ball (the part of the bone that is held within the hip joint) of the femoral bone (thigh bone) breaks off of the long part of the bone. The muscles contract and pull the whole leg up causing it to appear shortened as well as making it look like it is turned either inward or outward in an unnatural state. Other large deformities could include amputations (removal of a body extremity) and dislocations (separation of bones at the joint).

Fractures

A *fracture* is any injury in which a bony structure loses its functional ability. An open fracture is one in which the bone is exposed outside the body. Open fractures may or may not include a break in the bone but are often seen when a bone protrudes through the skin. Closed fractures are those that are not associated with any interruptions in the integrity of the skin. Complete fractures are seen when the "bone is broken all the way through" (McCance, Huether, Brashers, & Rote, 2010, p. 1560). An incomplete fracture is seen when the bone has a partial break in the structure.

THE INTEGUMENTARY SYSTEM

Skin, or the *integumentary* system, is a large organ that protects the delicate organs and systems of the body. The integumentary system plays a large role in regulating body temperature by sweating when hot or prickling when cold. Age affects skin;

the skin of a newborn is very flexible and durable, while the skin of an older adult is thin and more likely to tear. The skin has several layers. The outermost layer is the *epidermis* followed by the *dermis* and the deepest layer is the *subcutaneous tissue*.

Abrasion

When skin is rubbed off or scraped away, then an *abrasion* has occurred. This is a superficial (located near the surface of the skin) injury. A child who is running and falls on concrete typically has abrasions on their knees and palms as they skid across the rough surface and the skin is damaged. Abrasions may also occur in a more severe trauma such as a motor vehicle accident as the person is jostled on the inside of the car.

Decubiti

Decubiti or *pressure ulcers* are a breakdown in the skin due to external pressure exerted on the skin, typically on a bony area. They can also occur when friction is created between the skin and another surface. After a period of time, skin will breakdown and an ulcer will form. Older adults or people who are in beds or wheelchairs are more likely to develop these skin lesions. Decubiti are staged from *I to IV*. A *stage I* pressure ulcer is a *non-blanching* (does not change color if you press on the area with your finger) reddening of the skin. The color is different from the surrounding skin. *Stage II* is a shallow breakdown of the skin (dermis) and may be a blister or sloughing of the skin. Full thickness tissue loss that may extend to the subcutaneous fat (deeper fat layer of the skin) is staged as an *III decubiti*. Should bone, tendon, or muscle be exposed with full thickness tissue loss past the subcutaneous fat layer then the ulcer is deemed a *stage IV decubiti*.

Incisions and Lacerations

An *incision* is a purposeful interruption in the skin performed by a medical professional using a sharp cutting tool. Incisions are most often done during surgery to access an internal system. *Sutures* (stitches), staples, medical tape, or glue close incisions. A *closed* wound is either described as *approximated* or *non-approximated*. *Approximated* indicates that all edges are together and the wound is closed. The term *non-approximated* is used to indicate a wound has edges that are open. *Non-approximated* applies to the entire wound (completely open) or just a small portion of the wound is the result of problems with healing or *dehiscence* (force that reopened the wound).

Lacerations are a result of a trauma when a person is cut with a sharp instrument in a straight line *similar* to an incision. These cuts are uncontrolled and usually result in a longer healing process and more blood loss than an incision made by a surgeon.

Healthcare providers use a variety of terms to describe the amount, consistency, odor, and color of a wound's drainage. The medical terms used to describe *amount*,

TABLE 6.3 How to Describe Wound Drainage

Property	Range	Descriptors
Amount (volume)	From least to greatest	• Scant • Small • Moderate • Large • Copious
Consistency	From thinnest to thickest	• Thin • Thick • Purulent
Odor	Present or not present	No odor, foul odor
Color	Various shades	• Serous (straw colored or clear) • Serosanguineous (pink) • Sanguineous (bloody) or any other color (such as green)

or volume of drainage are, from least to greatest: *scant, small, moderate, large,* and *copious.* The terms used to describe consistency are thin, thick, and purulent. Odor is usually noted as either having no odor or having a foul odor, which indicates infection. Color is described as serous (straw colored and clear), serosanguineous (pink), sanguineous (bloody), or any other color such, as green (see Table 6.3).

Sometimes it is necessary to cover a wound to aid in proper healing. When a wound is covered, the materials used are called a *dressing.* Dressing supplies are varied and designed for specific purposes. Some dressings, such as abdominal pads (ABD's), have the primary purpose of absorbing drainage to wick moisture away from the wound to improve healing potential. Other dressings have *bacteriostatic* (prevent bacteria growth) properties. Common dressings include gauze wraps or pads usually referred to as 4×4s, packing material, non-stick pads, occlusive dressings, and hydrocolloid dressings.

Bruising

Bruising or *ecchymosis* (etchi-moh-sis) appears when there is a blood leakage from either superficial or deeper blood vessels between the layers of skin. Substantial bruising that forms a blood clot in the layers of skin is a *hematoma.* Hematomas are raised and swollen and usually reddened or purple at the time of injury. Bruising can be more superficial and generally fades from purple to green and then yellow as the body breaks down the accumulated blood during healing process.

Burns

Burns are classified in three categories and are classified by depth of the burn. These categories are *first degree, second degree,* and *third degree.* First degree burns damage only the first layer of skin called the epidermis; a common example of this type of burn is sunburn. Second degree burns destroy the epidermis and some of the dermis (layer of skin below the surface). These burns will generally have blisters and will either be red or white in color with a moist or dry surface depending on the depth of injury. Third degree burns show destruction of the epidermis, dermis, and some subcutaneous tissue. These burns appear as "white, cherry red or black and may appear as a hard leathery surface" (McCance et al., 2010, p. 1715).

Classification of Burns to the Skin		
Burn type	Damage	Presentation
First degree burns	Burn has damaged only the first layer, or epidermis	Example: Sunburn
Second degree burns	Burn destroys epidermis, some of the dermis.	Burns may have blisters and may be red or white, moist or dry surface depending on the depth of injury
Third degree burns	Epidermis, dermis, and some damage to subcutaneous tissue	Appears white, cherry red, or black; may have a hard leathery surface

Avulsions

An *avulsion* is created when a traumatic injury creates a "flap of skin." Avulsions are usually caused when something sharp cuts through the skin at a low angle and does not completely separate the flap from the body. These can be repaired with sutures after being cleaned thoroughly and treatment may include *prophylactic* (preventative) antibiotics.

Abbreviations and Other Common Terms   Abbreviations are commonly used, regardless of the professional context. As medical terminology tends to be quite lengthy at times, expediency in communication dictates that these are reduced in length. An SOS should familiarize themselves with abbreviations (typically acronyms) which are usually preferred over the actual word or phrase. Common abbreviations have been integrated into Appendix 1 of this book with terms and terminology. Such abbreviations aid the practitioner in both spoken and written communication.

CONCLUSION

This chapter provides an overview of medical terminology as it relates to the work of the SOS. By no means is this chapter comprehensive, but it should serve as a great icebreaker for the non-clinician working in simulation operations. As the SOS comes across new terminology and concepts, effort should be made to become acquainted with it and its implications for scenario design, programming, and simulator operation. With time, research, and exposure, the SOS can easily grasp the basics of medical terminology as it relates to simulation and its setup of realistic patient conditions.

REFERENCES

Atwood, S., Stanton, C., & Storey-Davenport, J. (2013). *Introduction to basic cardiac dysrhythmias*. Burlington, MA: James and Bartlett Learning.

Brooks, M. L., & Brooks, D. L. (2014). *Exploring medical language* (9th ed.). St. Louis, MO: Elsevier Mosby.

Chabner, D. (2015). *Medical terminology: A short course* (6th ed.). St Louis, MO: Elsevier Saunders.

Huether, S., & McCance, K. (2012). *Understanding pathophysiology* (5th ed.). St. Louis, MO: Elsevier Mosby.

McCance, K. L., Huether, S. E., Brashers, V. L., & Rote, N. S. (2010). *Pathophysiology: The biologic basis for disease in adults and children* (6th ed.). St. Louis, MO: Elsevier Mosby.

National Institute of Health. (2003). *NIH stroke scale*. Retrieved June 25, 2015, from http://www.ninds.nih.gov/doctors/nih_stroke_scale.pdf

Potter, P. A., Perry, A. G., Stockert, P. A., & Hall, A. M. (2012). *Fundamentals of nursing* (8th ed.). St. Louis, MO: Elsevier Mosby.

7

SIMULATION OPERATIONS, CURRICULUM INTEGRATION, AND PERFORMANCE IMPROVEMENT

TIMOTHY R. BROCK[1,2,3,4,5,6] AND MARY HOLTSCHNEIDER[7]

[1]*The Institute 4 Worthy Performance LLC, Winter Park, FL, USA*
[2]*The ROI Institute, Birmingham, AL, USA*
[3]*The Institute for Performance Improvement L3C, Chicago, IL, USA*
[4]*Full Sail University, Winter Park, FL, USA*
[5]*Franklin University, Columbus, OH, USA*
[6]*Webster University, St Louis, MO, USA*
[7]*Durham VA Medical Center, Durham, NC, USA*

INTRODUCTION

The great philosopher and futurist Bob Dylan once penned "The Times They Are A-Changin'" (1964). This is especially true for healthcare simulation operations and the Simulation Operations Specialist (SOS), an emerging healthcare profession. With the exception of space flight, simulation had humble beginnings in many professions. The developing healthcare SOS profession is traveling a similar trajectory as other simulation specialists from the military, aviation, nuclear power operations, law enforcement, firefighting, and space flight—to name a few.

While the history of simulation operations in each profession is well documented, this is not true for the evolution of the people who design and conduct the simulation sessions (Gantt, 2012). Individuals who do this work have varied backgrounds. Examples include simulation or simulator designers, instructors, individuals who train their replacements, or even warm bodies standing nearby. The same is true for

Healthcare Simulation: A Guide for Operations Specialists, First Edition.
Edited by Laura T. Gantt and H. Michael Young.
© 2016 John Wiley & Sons, Inc. Published 2016 by John Wiley & Sons, Inc.

healthcare simulation operations. A simple search of job descriptions yields positions for simulation specialists in technology, education, and training. Some job tasks overlap. Some are unique. Job descriptions can range from maintaining simulators to teaching/training others how to operate simulators, to (fill-in-the-blank) using a simulator. Job duties are driven by organizational needs, staffing limitations, and the workforce's ability to adapt.

Today, the healthcare simulation profession is sifting through the best blend of skill sets to determine if one outweighs others (i.e., clinician vs. technician and operator vs. educator/trainer). This sifting and sorting could create new, dedicated operations specialties within healthcare simulation. It is important to consider the SOS profession as an inclusive, emerging profession—not a mere job description—because simulation operations is not just about simulation duties or simulator technologies. Ultimately, simulation operations is about patient safety and quality care results. In other words, "do no harm."

Other chapters in this book address specific skills for simulation operations today. This chapter suggests a foundation for SOS professional development for individuals interested in creating a new, value-added, healthcare profession fit for the next generation of simulation operations. This evolving profession must provide healthcare performance improvement capabilities using simulation and simulation technologies as part of the larger healthcare provider or education systems.

THE MENTAL MODELS BEGIN AND END WITH SYSTEMS THINKING

To develop a mindset that focuses on results rather than the scenarios of discreet events of a simulation, there are three important conceptual models that can help position SOS professionals and their profession as more than just technology/educator/clinical people who use simulators. These models come from other high reliability organizations (HROs) that have integrated human performance architecture, safety management, risk management, and human error mitigation into their practices using simulation to prevent accidents and incidents. This HRO mindset begins and ends with systems thinking.

It is important to understand that a *systems* perspective differs from a *system* perspective. A *system* perspective begins with the larger system, or the sum total of the parts, whereas the *systems* perspective begins with the subsystems, or the parts of the system (Kaufman, Oakley-Brown, Watkins, & Lee, 2003). The SOS starts with the human performance subsystem.

Just as systems thinking helps the simulation technician operate and troubleshoot standalone and integrated simulation technologies, the systems thinking perspective will help the SOS offer important perspectives and capabilities for creating and sustaining high reliability healthcare systems. Systems thinking helps the mindful observer recognize overlooked patterns and details that affect human performance as part of a learning organization (Senge, 1990). This includes using simulation to assess, improve, and sustain the performance of practicing healthcare professionals. The same is true of education programs preparing students to perform at acceptable levels of competence during their instructional programs and after graduation.

This systems thinking perspective forces the SOS professional, as well as the other simulation team members and stakeholders,[1] to consider the larger system that the simulation program affects. This includes the other side of how the larger healthcare or education system affects what occurs during the simulation. This systems perspective increases everyone's systemic awareness of the "multiplicity of relationships" that can affect the simulation design and how simulation accomplishments will affect the larger system (MacDonald, McDowell, Siegel, & DeLeon, 2014, p. 275). The goal is to successfully integrate the simulation as part of the larger healthcare provider or education system (Coleman, Menaker, & Murawski, 2000).

Mental Model 1: Establishing the Value of Simulation Operations

It is important for SOS professionals to understand they are an important part of a "means to an end" in the Human Performance Value Stream. This is true whether using simulation to teach, design, or test human performance or to integrate technologies to maximize their value. In healthcare, the end is delivering safe, quality care expected by the patient and the public. Simulation is a means used to close knowledge and skill gaps required to achieve these desired human and organizational results. Knowing and proving the value of the SOS profession in this Human Performance Value Stream is foundational to establishing a new, respected healthcare profession.

The Human Performance Value Stream provides a clear conceptual model to help frame how to think through a *systematic process* to help healthcare educators and performance improvement professionals analyze performance deficiencies and opportunities. This model is derived from multiple theorists and models such as the front-end analysis performance chain (Harless, 1998), behavior engineering model (Gilbert, 1996), six boxes approach (Binder, 2007), and the organizational elements model (Kaufman & Guerra-Lopez, 2013).

Figure 7.1 illustrates how the Human Performance Value Stream begins with selecting the right people with the right competence (knowledge, skills, and attributes), capabilities (ability to learn and improve), and commitment (attitudes/motivation) to do a job. The organization provides them with the resources required to do that job and to grow into higher responsible positions. They then use these resources to perform job tasks. Their task behaviors produce accomplishments—results or outcomes. These accomplishments are what determine whether the organization achieves its goals to fulfill its reason for existing. Where does simulation for education or performance improvement fall in this Human Performance Value Stream? To answer that question, this section will look at each phase of this process.

People   Selecting the right people for the right positions is the essential first step to achieve organizational results. This is true for hiring, onboarding, qualifying, retaining, and promoting people at all levels. Effective organizations are about competent people performing defined tasks to competency standards. Hiring prerequisites are

---

[1] A stakeholder is someone who has a vested interest in the valued accomplishments produced by simulation operations and their resulting workplace, organizational, and societal impact.

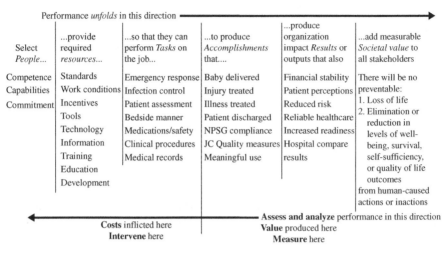

Performance *unfolds* in this direction →					
Select *People...*	...provide required resources...	...so that they can perform *Tasks* on the job...	...to produce *Accomplishments* that....	...produce organization impact *Results* or outputs that also	...add measurable *Societal value* to all stakeholders
Competence Capabilities Commitment	Standards Work conditions Incentives Tools Technology Information Training Education Development	Emergency response Infection control Patient assessment Bedside manner Medications/safety Clinical procedures Medical records	Baby delivered Injury treated Illness treated Patient discharged NPSG compliance JC Quality measures Meaningful use	Financial stability Patient perceptions Reduced risk Reliable healthcare Increased readiness Hospital compare results	There will be no preventable: 1. Loss of life 2. Elimination or reduction in levels of well-being, survival, self-sufficiency, or quality of life outcomes from human-caused actions or inactions

← **Costs** inflicted here
Intervene here

Assess and analyze performance in this direction →
Value produced here
Measure here

FIGURE 7.1   Human Performance Value Stream. Reproduced with permission from The Institute 4 Worthy Performance, LLC.

defined by job task accomplishment requirements. It is crucial to hire the right person, or educate the right entry-level candidate, to do a job to a predefined level of proficiency. These prerequisites can involve experience, academic degrees, credentials, and even intangibles a resume cannot capture. Hiring mistakes are costly for the organization and for the people hired to do something they cannot, or will not, do.

Simulation does, or can, play a role in educating, screening, or assessing people and teams. This curriculum and assessment can be (i) part of a degree program where simulation is integrated into the curriculum, (ii) during the hiring process, or (iii) in team development training. The SOS professional will play an important role in designing, developing, and delivering effective simulation-based learning experiences and assessments.

Resources   Organizations cannot expect the people they hire to do their job right the first time if they do not give them the resources needed for competent performance. Education programs have the same obligation to give their faculty/students what they need to effectively teach/learn and to perform competently. Again, this applies to all levels of the healthcare and education organizational structures. Tools, technology, a safe work/learning environment, performance guidance (i.e., policies, procedures, and standards), incentives, and professional development opportunities to stay relevant and promotable (i.e., training and education) are just a few examples.

Providing the right resources enables people to learn, perform, and improve. Not providing these resources creates barriers to optimal performance. Simulation operations can serve a vital developmental role with staff and student education and training and help refine policies, procedures, and processes to improve individual, team, and organizational performance. Simulation operations professionals can also support developmental research and systems integration efforts to find ways to improve the resources people require to do their jobs and uncover barriers that prevent them from performing to standard (Fig. 7.1). The SOS professional who thinks from a Human Performance Value Stream perspective makes sure simulation events or projects include resources that accurately reflect the real-world work environment.

To put this in instructional design terms, resources define two of the three parts of a Criterion Objective listed in Table 7.1 (Dick, Carey, & Carey, 2014; Mager, 1997; Noe, 2013). The same is true for objectives written using Gagne's five-part format[2] (Gagne, Briggs, & Wagner, 1992; Handshaw, 2014) and the SMART[3] method.

Tasks   People perform tasks when they do their jobs. Tasks have a beginning and an end. Tasks are the third part of a Criterion Objective, which is defined in Table 7.2.

There are different ways to classify tasks. It is important for the SOS professional to know the difference between the types of tasks because they affect how simulations are conducted. One way is to classify tasks as either *procedural* or *principal-based* (Clark, 1999a; Foshay, Silber, & Stelnicki, 2003). These two classifications of tasks are also identified as *near-transfer* and *far-transfer tasks* (Clark, 1999b; Noe, 2013).

There are two types of *procedural* tasks—linear and branching. Linear procedural tasks involve observable steps that, when followed, produce an accomplishment

TABLE 7.1   Criterion Objective Conditions and Standards Definitions

Objective Element	Definition	Examples
Condition(s)	To write condition(s), specify what the learner is GIVEN to perform the action in a job-like setting. Describes the conditions for performance. "What is presented to the learner to perform the action?"	• Data • Environmental conditions • Equipment • Job aids • Location • Special instructions • Technical references • Tools
Standard(s)	To write standard(s), specify HOW WELL learner needs to perform the task or performance behavior in a job-like setting. Describes the output or outcome of the performance action. "How well must the learner perform the action?"	• Completeness • Accuracy • Standard operating procedure (SOP) • No error • Time requirements • Rate requirements • Amount of supervision • Quality indicators

[2] Gagne's five parts of a learning objective are (1) situation (the stimulus for performing a task), (2) learning capability (the action verb for the task), (3) object (the object of the task), (4) action (how the task is performed), and (5) tools/constraints (what the performer requires to perform the task and what constraints exist, such as time or level of proficiency).

[3] SMART represents specific, measurable, attainable/achievable, results-focused/realistic, and time-focused/bound.

TABLE 7.2   Criterion Objective Task or Performance Definition

Objective Element	Definition	Examples
Task	To write a task or performance behavior, specify what the learner is expected to DO after the simulation on the job. Describes the action or behavior. "What is the learner expected to do?"	Use action verbs that are: • Measurable • Observable • Specific • Has a beginning and an end • Verifiable • Reliable (not prone to varying interpretation)

(i.e., result or outcome). Branching (or decision-based) procedural tasks can take one or more linear procedural paths following observable steps. The path taken depends upon a criterion used to make a decision. One approach is the IF:THEN algorithm (i.e., IF this happens, THEN do this). Procedures are done the same way every time the task is performed. Simulation can easily replicate them in a job-like setting. They are called near-transfer tasks because the steps are performed during the simulations the same way they are on the job. The simulation can replicate (or get close/near to) how the task is performed in every situation.

Principal-based tasks are situational and require judgment to apply guidelines. How the guidelines are applied depends on the situation, which typically includes unpredictable responses as events unfold. There is no one right way to perform the principle-based task. The guidelines, when properly applied, should produce the desired task accomplishment. These tasks are called *far-transfer* because the simulation cannot replicate every situation the student will encounter on the job to learn how to best apply the guidelines in those situations. Instead, different circumstances are presented and the student develops self-management skills to determine how to apply the guidelines in unique, different situations.

Tasks are also referred to as *hard* and *soft* skills. Hard skills are technical. Soft skills are conceptual and interpersonal (e.g., reasoning, logic, communication, leadership, management, and social) and are harder to train (Hale, 2012).

Regardless of how they are categorized, tasks produce results or outputs that are considered accomplishments. Simulation's role at this level is indirect and diagnostic. Did the simulation improve the performance of the individuals or team as intended? In addition, can simulation reproduce the work environment and the given resources to diagnose workplace performance deficiencies to find the right remedy?

Accomplishments   An accomplishment is a measurable consequence of behavior. Behavior is a means to that end. A useful memory aid to help distinguish between the two is "behavior is something you take with you, accomplishment is something you leave behind" (Gilbert & Gilbert, 1989, p. 3). In addition, the affected stakeholders must value an accomplishment. If it is not valued, it is simply an output or result (Addison, Haig, & Kearney, 2009). From the Human Performance Value Stream perspective, accomplishments occur when the right people with the right resources are doing the right task, the right way, the first time.

Mager (1997) illustrated how to distinguish between achieving an accomplishment (performing to a criterion) and achieving a desired passing score typically associated with instruction. If one performs a 10-step procedure to make coffee but misses the step to put the coffee into the coffeemaker, some can argue that this is a passing score for completing the task (9 out of 10 steps correct yields a 90% score). However, the result was hot water and not coffee. This is not the desired, or valued, accomplishment. Both healthcare education and healthcare provider organizations want the accomplishments.

This is where the Human Performance Value Stream perspective establishes the value of simulation. Simulation operations is about valued accomplishments and impact results, not about simulations. Simulation operations can replicate the work environment to allow for learning or assessment. This assessment allows for evidence-based decisions about an individual or team's competence to perform a task or accomplish a required result.

When developing or delivering simulation, what accomplishments do the stakeholders and the participants[4] expect? A key tactic for the success of performance improvement and learning solutions that include simulation is to earn the buy-in of all stakeholders and align expectations by seeking as many key stakeholder voices as possible during the design phase (MacDonald et al., 2014). The learning objectives define the required accomplishment(s) and create a contract for ensuring the stakeholders, learning/performance improvement team, and simulation team start with the same end in mind (Handshaw, 2014).

Finally, the objectives are the first criterion used to determine the right methods and media for the simulation (Dick et al., 2014; Foster, Melon, & Phillips, 2007; US Department of Defense, 2001). Simulation media examples include part-task trainers, standardized (or simulated) patients, virtual reality, serious games, computer-based simulation, in situ, manikin-based, or blended (or hybrid) simulation.

Results The Human Performance Value Stream continues its focus on establishing value. Every organization establishes measurable impact goals to achieve defined results and outcomes. Organizational leaders use impact goals to determine where to dedicate limited resources. Often, the decisions about whether or not to initiate or to continue funding simulation are based on perceived and demonstrated value that simulation operations add to the organization.

Why is this important? As with everything, we must measure and evaluate the balance between cost and value, or return on investment (ROI). The "no margin, no mission" phrase used by executives applies to both for-profit and not-for-profit organizations. Healthcare executives are now asking hard questions and want proof

---

[4] A participant can be a stakeholder but a stakeholder may not be a participant. A nurse supervisor who sends a nurse for training using simulation is the stakeholder, while the nurse is the simulation participant and a stakeholder. The executives who pay for the simulations are stakeholders and not a simulation participant.

about the value of programs and projects to include ROI (Buzachero, Phillips, Phillips, & Phillips, 2013). This includes efforts to improve human performance. Gilbert (1996) first linked human performance improvement to cost and value. Phillips (1997) integrated ROI into Kirkpatrick's (1994) four levels of evaluation to provide tangible economic evidence that executives want to prove the value of non-capital investments. More important than a formula, it is this cost/value balance that establishes the worth of something and has Human Performance Value Stream implications.

Value is both tangible and intangible. Healthcare and simulation program administrators want to know what they are getting from their investment. Even more, they want to know the *tangible* and *intangible* results that were achieved and also have proof that simulation operations is not taking credit for improvements produced by another means. Figure 7.2 indicates how more healthcare administrators are already transitioning the focus from "activities" to "results" (Buzachero et al., 2013). This accountability evolution transitions from *data* to *meaningful data* (i.e., both tangible and intangible evidence) that is credible and defendable.

If simulation is not adding value or making a patient safety/quality care difference, why continue funding it? Justifying the expense of simulation is a challenge when others are competing for the same limited dollars. Remember where value is established in the Human Performance Value Stream (see Fig. 7.1).

For some, the relevance of this accountability evolution may seem remote. Regardless, this higher level of accountability is inevitable. It is better to prepare now for this coming value-based accountability standard rather than wait for an executive request to justify simulation expenses. If SOS skills are limited to setting up and running simulation events, cost-cutting measures can result in staffing decisions to ask others, like nurse educators, to pick up the duties of downsized SOS positions.

Societal Value   Healthcare providers and educators have a social contract with the public to do no harm. The *societal value* phase establishes the ideal outcomes desired by a healthcare organization that are achieved through the human performance chain.

Term	Issue
Show me!	Collect impact data
Show me the money!	And convert data to money
Show me the real money!	And isolate the effects of the project
Show me the real money, and make me believe it's a great investment!	And compare the money to the cost of the project

FIGURE 7.2   Accountability evolution. Reproduced with permission from The ROI Institute, Inc.

This ideal vision establishes the common purpose that all organizational subsystems must work toward to add value. This phase reflects the strategic thinking level of the organizational elements model (Kaufman, 2000). This strategic thinking level establishes the vital and measurable healthcare *system* perspective that aligns all of its *subsystems* that are critical for sustained organizational success. Its primary focus is on "creating the world we want for future generations" (Kaufman & Guerra-Lopez, 2013, p. 30). The challenge for SOS professionals is to continuously position simulation operations, through the human performance value chain, as a value-added human performance improvement subsystem rather than as an activity-based cost center.

Mental Model 2: The Role of Simulation Operations

Simulation operations delivers value at the *accomplishment* and *results* phases and serve different roles within organizations (see Fig. 7.1). The value simulation creates depends upon the role it serves in the healthcare system.

Dr. Jennifer Arnold, the Medical Director of Pediatric Simulation Center and a Neonatologist at Texas Children's Newborn Center, proposes a valuable framework for simulation that identifies five roles. She describes these as the "Arms of Simulation" (Arnold, 2012), which are listed as follows:

1. Training and clinical rehearsal
2. Education and advocacy
3. Research and development
4. Assessment of competence (high stakes)
5. Improvement in patient safety and quality care

The Society for Simulation in Healthcare (SSH) defines healthcare simulation as a "range of activities that share a broad, similar purpose—to improve the safety, effectiveness, and efficiency of healthcare services" (2014). SSH then offers a similar list of roles for healthcare simulation. Listed below are the activities advocated by SSH with a brief explanation of each one. To read the full description of each role, see www.ssih.org/About-Simulation.

1. Simulation operations—a bridge between safe, real-life learning and safe, quality patient care
2. Simulation-based assessments—both "low stakes" learning for improvement and "high stakes" testing to determine competency
3. Simulation-based research—increasing knowledge and understanding to improve training, evaluation, and design of systems
4. Systems integration—the integration of simulation into institutional healthcare training and delivery systems

The Institute 4 Worthy Performance developed an integrated framework that modifies the roles of simulation identified by Arnold (2012) and SSH (2014). This

Purpose

• Patient safety and quality care

Practices

• Education

• Training and clinical rehearsal

• Competence assessment
  (low and high stakes)

• Systems performance integration

Partnership

• Safe, effective, efficient healthcare services

• Learning healthcare system

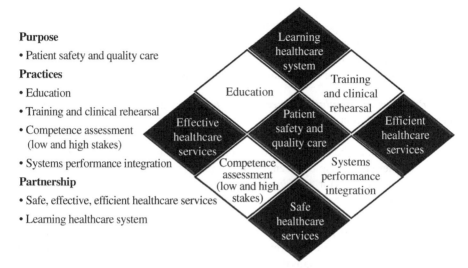

FIGURE 7.3 The nine roles of simulation operations. Reproduced with permission from The Institute 4 Worthy Performance LLC.

framework establishes nine roles of simulation operations. Each role supports the Human Performance Value Stream introduced at Figure 7.1. These nine roles are organized into a 3×3 diamond grid represented in Figure 7.3. This framework also indicates how these nine roles are classified into three categories: *purpose*, *practices*, and *partnership*.

At the center of this framework is the *purpose* of healthcare simulation operations (and healthcare operations)—patient safety and quality care. Four *practices* border the four sides of the *purpose* rhombus and represent the means to the end where value is established (see Fig. 7.1). These four *practices* are (1) education, (2) training and clinical rehearsal, (3) competence assessment (low and high stakes), and (4) systems performance integration. Each of these roles fit into the human performance systems framework represented in the Human Performance Value Stream. *Practices* (in white in Fig. 7.3) occur when performing tasks.

The *partnership* roles complete the 3×3 diamond grid and identify critical impact goals—a learning healthcare system that delivers safe (do no harm), effective (do what's right), and efficient (do it well) healthcare services. *Partnership* and *purpose* (in black in Fig. 7.3) are the results of these *practices*. The outcomes of the *practices* and *partnerships* fulfill the *purpose*.

The Purpose of Simulation Operations This 3×3 diamond grid establishes the *purpose* of healthcare simulation operations as patient safety and quality care at the center of the model that all other roles revolve around. This purpose matches, or aligns with, the purpose of healthcare system operations represented by the Human Performance Value Stream (Fig. 7.1). It establishes the measurable value of education and performance improvement programs, projects, or initiatives at the *results* phases (see Fig. 7.1). If a simulation does not directly support improving or sustaining patient safety and quality care, the activity is suspect and risk being perceived as not value-added in the Human Performance Value Stream. One should note that the purpose of simulation as defined by this model differs from the purpose of simulation advocated by SSH. The 3×3 diamond grid reclassifies the SSH's purpose of simulation as three *partnership* roles.

The Practices of Simulation Operations   *Practices* are specific activities where healthcare simulation operations are used to achieve its patient safety and quality care accomplishments. *Practices* are found at the *people* and *resources* phases, the first two phases, of the Human Performance Value Stream (see Fig. 7.1). One could argue that there is overlap between the four *practices*. However, these four *practices* provide a framework for *thinking* and a focus for *application*. Dissecting these perceived overlaps is beyond the scope of this chapter.

- Education—This *practice* is associated with *select people* (Fig. 7.1), the first phase of the Human Performance Value Stream. Not many professions have academic degree programs directly attached to workplaces equipping them with a stream of potential employees. One example is teaching hospitals and other healthcare systems with relationships with colleges and universities offering healthcare degree programs. The healthcare industry is uniquely positioned to integrate simulation into its academic degree programs to minimize the healthcare provider preparation-to-practice gap that delays declaring a new hire "patient-ready." Various types of simulations and simulator devices or platforms offering different levels of fidelity (realism) and technical complexity are becoming more common in academic curricula. In addition, state accrediting agencies recognize the effectiveness of simulation as a competency-based learning medium that can replace clinical learning time (Hayden, Smiley, Alexander, Kardong-Edgren, & Jeffries, 2014). Not only can instructionally sound simulation allow healthcare students (and professionals) to practice and learn without any real-time risk to patient safety or quality care, but this medium can, if used appropriately, decrease the time and cost to achieve competence. Added-value simulation in healthcare curricula directly influences the quality of graduates (Hayden et al., 2014). As the number of healthcare education simulation programs grow, so will the demand for credentialed healthcare SOS professionals who know how to add measurable value within the Human Performance Value Stream.

- Training and Clinical Rehearsal—This *practice* is related to improving and sustaining the proficiency of people on the job. Simulation operations can play a critical role in improving the performance of individuals and teams. Simulations add value to healthcare delivery systems by improving and sustaining patient safety and quality care accomplishments. The perception that years of experience somehow predict a level of competence is a false premise (Bond & Cooper, 2006; Brock, 2007; Gilbert, 1996). In addition, staffing challenges are overworking healthcare professionals, allowing knowledge and skill decay to occur over time (Arthur, Bennett, Stanush, & McNelly, 1998). Other HROs build recurring training using simulation into the schedules of their workforce to validate competence and prevent decay. Aviation, nuclear power operations, the military, and space exploration are four HROs that come to mind. This list should include healthcare professions as well. Knowledge and skill decay (aka "use it or lose it") is a reality. Physicians and nurses returning to civilian hospitals from lengthy military assignments in war zones know this decay exists (Rush, 2013; Skinner, 2014). Simulation offers great benefits when learning new skills, sustaining these skills, and refreshing skills when returning to a position. In addition, clinical rehearsal of procedures to maintain proficiency, such as mock codes, is also an important application of simulation operations.

- Competence Assessment (High and Low Stakes)—Assessing competence must include both the new hire and current workforce populations. Simulation-based assessment seeks to replicate the work environment as closely as necessary to determine whether an individual or team possesses the level of competence required to provide safe, quality patient care. This type of assessment currently occurs in aviation, nuclear power, the military, first responders, and in space exploration for routine and emergency situations. Low stakes assessments focus on determining if learning is occurring and performance is proficient or improving. High stakes assessments determine competence. Failing to demonstrate competence during a high stakes assessment can result in someone or a team losing a credential, license, or certification. For example, in the military, if a flight crew or a missile launch crew fails to perform at a specified level of competency, they are decertified and must requalify after completing training designed to remedy their knowledge and skill gap. The healthcare industry is moving toward using simulation to assess competence. The role of the healthcare SOS is critical to ensure that simulation events occur at the right fidelity to reflect the workplace environment, precisely as scripted, and to standards.

- Systems Performance Integration—This practice is a blend of Arnold's Research and Development (R&D) and SSH's Systems Integration. R&D seeks to change or maintain the healthcare system and subsystems to find better ways to improve value stream performance efficiencies and effectiveness without sacrificing quality. The same is true for systems integration. However, rather than focus on how to integrate simulation into the institutional healthcare training and delivery systems advocated by SSH, this practice is about routinely using simulation operations to integrate the subsystems to change or maintain the healthcare system. Examples are mechanical systems (i.e., technologies), business systems (i.e., workflow or patient care processes), and human performance systems (discussed later in this chapter). This practice directly supports the taxonomy of performance (Swanson, 2007) represented in Table 7.3.

Credentialed SOS professionals will find opportunities to make even greater contributions to the accomplishments achieved and goals attained by helping healthcare systems use simulation appropriately as a means to an end when considering the Human Performance Value Stream framework.

The Partnerships for Simulation Operations The Human Performance Value Stream clearly indicates that simulation operations do not occur in a vacuum. The

TABLE 7.3   Taxonomy of Performance

Changing the System	
Invent	Produce a new method, process, device, or system from study or experimentation.
Improve	Advance an existing method, process, device, or system to a better state or quality.
Maintaining the System	
Troubleshoot	Locate and eliminate sources of trouble in an existing method, process, device, or system.
Operate	Run or control the functioning of a method, process, device, or system.
Understand	Comprehend the language, sounds, form, or symbols of an existing method, process, device, or system.

beginning of this chapter made the point that healthcare simulation operations is "an important part of a means to an end." This requires first defining the "end" the stakeholders expect the simulation to produce in return for their funding investment. This includes the "accomplishments" (or leading performance indicators) and "impact results" (or lagging performance indicators). The SOS professional does not define this, the customers and stakeholders[5] of the simulation do. However, the SOS professional must demonstrate an understanding of the big picture, or Human Performance Value Stream perspective, to help these customers and stakeholders achieve the results they want simulation operations to deliver. This involves *partnerships*, the four outermost roles of simulation operations, as seen in Figure 7.3.

- Effective Healthcare Services—Through the preceding four *practice* roles, SOS professionals should help determine the best clinical care procedures, practices, principles, and processes to deliver the safest, high quality patient care possible. By partnering with simulation stakeholders and learning what accomplishments the simulations must equip people to produce, the SOS professional can dialogue with stakeholders and SOS community-of-practice professionals to help develop and deliver effective healthcare services.
- Efficient Healthcare Services—SOS professionals must have a value-focused mindset when creating simulations and observing simulation events. They are in a unique position to observe various professions using simulation and learn different techniques and practices to achieve desired outcomes and practices. They may then use this cross-pollination position to introduce customers to

[5]A customer is a type of stakeholder. While both have a vested interest in the valued accomplishments of the simulation, the customer is the direct recipient of the simulation results. The customer focus is on job/learning performance accomplishments and leading performance indicators. Stakeholders realize the results or outcomes as the improved job/leaning performance (a properly prepared patient for surgery/met performance objectives) or as downstream lagging performance indicators (lower readmission rates due to infections/prepared for next curriculum phase). Stakeholders are affected by the cost and benefits of the effectiveness of the simulation to achieve one of the four practices and the purpose of simulation operations.

different perspectives and approaches to effectively and efficiently get the desired results during simulation operations. By making connections between stakeholders, customers, and peers, the SOS can create a culture of collaboration for delivering simulations that produce results.

- Safe Healthcare Services—It is sad to hear people correctly relate data that support the claim the hospitals pose a danger to patients. "Do no harm" is a simple phrase that too often seems to have gotten lost in today's healthcare delivery systems. Instructionally sound and accomplishment-focused simulations can allow participants to make mistakes without harming patients as well as to identify deficient procedures, practices, principles, and processes. The SOS professional will witness simulations that assist in identifying these deficiencies and become an oracle for what works and what works better when helping healthcare educators and trainers during the simulation scenario design, development, implementation, evaluation phases.

- Learning Healthcare System—Neither the Arnold framework (2012) nor the SSH definition of simulation (2014) includes this role. Rather than listing the attributes of a learning organization to explain this role (see Senge (1990) for this explanation), imagine three possibilities. First, imagine being a part of a healthcare organization where simulation operations is considered a valued *partner* by the education, performance improvement, and quality care teams. Then, imagine the quality care and safety lessons learned from the four *practices* of simulation operations being shared with these *partners* for meeting or improving human and organization performance. Finally, imagine simulation operations as a key component of discussions between executives and healthcare educators/practitioners to educate or prepare people to perform their jobs more effectively, efficiently, and safely. Simulation operations is where significant, if not critical, learning and improving healthcare provider proficiency can occur. Simulation can assist in the validation of undergraduate curriculum as well as with competency and readiness assessments in the professional theatre.

Mental Model 3: The Focus of Simulation Operations

Viewing human performance from a *systems* perspective provides a valuable framework the SOS professional can use to apply the Human Performance Value Stream framework within each element of the 3×3 roles of simulation model. This perspective looks at how performance unfolds from a human performance system perspective at a more detailed level the Human Performance Value Stream perspective provides. It is an extension of the early work referenced for Human Performance Value Stream to include the performance analysis flowchart model (Mager & Piper, 1997), performance diagnosis matrix (Swanson, 2007), the human performance system model (Brethower, 1967; Rummler & Brache, 1995), and the culpability decision tree (Reason, 1997).

The performance of people delivering a product or service is the core of the Human Performance Value Stream. People perform work tasks to produce accomplishments. This is true at every level of an organization. Technology, processes, and other resources are provided to people to help them increase their capabilities to perform those work tasks the *right* way the *first* time. When something goes wrong, the default first response is to blame people under the category of human error. Someone either did something wrong or should have foreseen the error to prevent it.

Healthcare looks to other industries as benchmarks for simulation and clinical operations to minimize human error when providing patient care. The increasing push for using checklists comes from their demonstrated value in aviation. Other important lessons learned come from research of, and by, HROs (e.g., aviation and nuclear power operations) where human error can have catastrophic outcomes. Their incident and accident studies seek to uncover underlying causes. Too often, the findings are erroneously attributed to human error.

Research by Perrow (1984), Reason (1999), and the *Institute for Nuclear Power Operations* (INPO) (US Department of Energy, 2009) on accident and incident investigations indicates that 80% of accident and incident causes were attributed to human error and 20% were attributed to mechanical failure. However, when researchers conducted a more in-depth diagnosis of human error, 30% of these human errors where caused by individual mistakes and 70% were caused by latent organizational weaknesses. Latent organizational weaknesses are unknown human errors in a system from the past that do not surface until triggered by another event (Reason, 1999). Analysis of the British Petroleum Deepwater Horizon incident at the Gulf of Mexico produced similar findings (Hubbard & Embrey, 2010). Figure 7.4, adapted from the US Department of Energy *Human Performance Improvement Handbook* (2009), graphically illustrates this more in-depth understanding of human error research.

INPO reports that investigations of the nuclear power plant community's significant events occurring between 1995 and 1999 indicated that three out of every four events were caused by human error. Even more, the Nuclear Regulatory Agency reports that human error was the critical factor in 81% (24 out of 26) of significant events where fuel was damaged while in the reactor. This report revealed "the risk is in the people—the way they are trained, their level of professionalism and performance, and the way they are managed" (US Department of Energy, 2009,

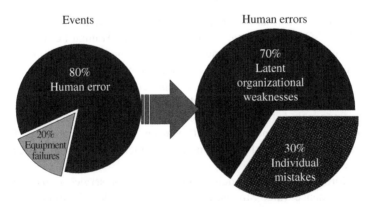

FIGURE 7.4   Human error vs. latent organizational weaknesses root causes.

pp. 1–10). In response to these findings, the Department of Energy, in collaboration with INPO, instituted proactive human performance measures, like the ones presented in this chapter, to prevent human error.

Rummler succinctly identified the root cause of most human error during the mid-1960s with the statement, "If you pit a good performer against a bad system, the system will win every time" (Rummler, 2004, p. xviii; Rummler & Brache, 1992).

What does this mean to the SOS professional? Today, probably not much. However, what is done today creates the future. Growing a reputation as a performance improvement partner whose expertise is simulation operations rather than as a simulation technology technician, operator educator, or trainer will establish greater value and respect from healthcare administrators, patient safety, quality, risk management, governing bodies, and, ideally, patients who focus on results and outcomes. The key is to ask the right questions to determine root causes of human error undermining the human performance system. The seminal book, *To Err is Human: Building a Safer Healthcare System* (Institute of Medicine, 1999), confirms this issue is relevant to healthcare and the importance of the Human Performance Value Stream framework.

A helpful way for the SOS professional to sort and assemble this Human Performance Value Stream perspective is to look at requests for simulation support from a human performance systems perspective. This involves applying the elements of a system to people performing a task (typical scenarios are not about a single task, but about the critical thinking that occurs in that context), which is what simulation is designed to instruct and improve. A system typically is composed of an input, process, output, and consequence. Figure 7.5 shows how Rummler and Brache (1995) changed the process element to performer and added consequences after the output to become the source of feedback. Viewing human performance as a system gives a very different lens for diagnosing performance deficiencies and creating realistic simulation situations and environments because it focuses on what people need to do their job tasks. This perspective also aligns with the elements involved with writing effective simulation learning objectives. This perspective also helps those seeking simulation support to uncover latent organizational weaknesses as well as individual/team performance deficiencies the simulation must address to achieve the desired outcome.

Figure 7.5 shows how these five interdependent system variables affect human performance on-the-job and during simulations. This human performance system framework aligns well with the Human Performance Value Stream framework (see

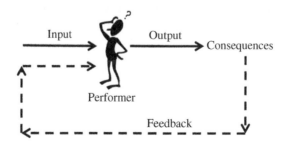

FIGURE 7.5   The elements of a human performance system.

Fig. 7.1). The *performer* clearly represents the first phase of having the right people with the right competencies performing job *tasks*. The *output* represents the *accomplishments* from performing the *tasks*. *Inputs, consequences*, and *feedback* are part of the *resources* organizations must provide its workforce to perform their assigned job *tasks* to an appropriate standard.

Output   Outputs produce the accomplishments that justify the reason a position exists in the organization. *Outputs* focus on defining what Rummler and Brache call performance specifications (1995). Effective learning objectives establish the performance specifications that should mirror task accomplishments if they are written correctly. Each *output* is related directly to learning objectives. Output-focused questions that require answers are: *Do performance specifications (or standards) exist and are they current and accurate?*; *Is performance measured and are measurements based on task performance?*; *Are the measurements objective?*; and *Does the performer consider the performance specification attainable?*

If people do not know what is expected of them or do not believe they can do the task, they likely fail. The time to ask these questions is when designing a simulation event. If a simulation participant seems uncertain or hesitant about what to do during a simulation, is it an *output* or performance standard problem? Looking for and asking the right questions about *output* issues can uncover barriers to performance that reside outside of the individual. These are organizational support deficiencies. It is unreasonable to hold people accountable for failing to meet standards during a simulation, or on the job, if the standards do not exist, are not known to the performers, or are unattainable by the performers. No one in the simulation community is better positioned to consider these issues during the planning and design phases than the SOS professional.

Input   The second variable that affects human performance is the *input* the performers receive to perform the work task. This is also called task performance support by Rummler and Brache (1995). Inputs are likewise directly related to the learning objectives. They involve what the performer requires to start and perform a task. For example, does the performer know when to start a task by recognizing a trigger event (such as an assignment or request to do something with clear direction and a sensory signal) and how to respond to the "trigger"? Do the performer and supervisor agree on the performance specification and output? Can the task be done without interference from other tasks or barriers to performance? Is the job task design and workflow logical? Is the performer provided job/performance support aids? Is the performer provided adequate resources to achieve the required outcomes (time, tools, staff, information, etc.)?

These questions seem straightforward. Yet, they are often overlooked, even when designing and conducting simulations. Each phase of this model is essential for the SOS professional to consider to capitalize on the organization's investment in simulation operations. This human performance system model applies to every position at all levels of an organization.

Performer   The next variable is about the people performing the task. *Performers* convert *inputs* into *outputs*. The *performer* variable relates to whether or not people know what is expected of them, have the knowledge, skills, attitudes, and attributes (i.e., mental, physical, and emotional competencies) to perform the required tasks. Four questions people often ask themselves when asked or directed to perform a task: (1) "Do I know what is expected of me?"; (2) "Can I do it?"; (3) "Will I be given what I need to do it?"; and (4) "Do I want to do it?". The answers to these questions are where simulation can have significant, direct influence. Simulation can play a major role with diagnostic, formative, summative, and high stakes competency assessments to uncover the answers to all four questions.

Consequences   Both positive and negative *consequences* can result from the outputs produced by a performer. The *performer* determines whether a *consequence* is positive or negative. What happens if someone does or does not do a task to achieve an expected "standard"? Is it worth the effort? If they do not do it right, does it matter? Does the organizational system reward desired behavior in a way that makes the *performer* value it thereby encouraging the desired behavior? If the *consequences* do not occur in a timely manner, the desired behavior will likely decrease or stop because it seems what they are doing does not matter. During simulation, are the *consequences* of *performer* actions reflective of what happen in the workplace? Do they support and reward the desired performance? Are they timely, meaningful, and desired by the *performer*? Senge sums the importance of paying attention to and learning from consequences by stating, "Herein lies the core learning dilemma that confronts organizations: We learn best from experience but we never directly experience the consequences of many of our most important decisions" (1990, p. 23).

Feedback   *Performers* need *feedback* to let them know how they are doing. *Feedback* comes in different forms. For example, *performers* can receive *feedback* to actions they take while performing the task so they can adjust their actions accordingly. *Performers* can also receive *feedback* about their behavior or their *accomplishments* after completing tasks from reports (e.g., error rates and productivity), and comments from customers, supervisors, or colleagues, and evaluations. Feedback systems are typically neglected as a formal part of a human performance system. *Performers* are expected to monitor their own performance. Corrective or affirmative feedback from their supervisors occurs once or twice a year during their performance appraisals.

It is important for *performers* to receive delayed *feedback* about their performance in a timely manner so they can make adjustments. It is also important for the *feedback* to focus on performance (rather than personality) and come from someone who matters to the *performer*. In addition, the *feedback* must be relevant, accurate, specific, and easy to understand. *Feedback* is more than a debrief at the end of the simulation session. First, real-time *feedback* must also occur while the human is interacting with the larger system during simulation. For example, if a *performer* is taking an action and is not getting the intended response from the patient or monitoring systems, the simulation systems provides *feedback* on those actions that the *performer* must recognize, interpret, and then adapt their behavior to take corrective action.

Rummler and Brache state, from a human performance system perspective, that "the quality of outputs is a function of inputs, performers, consequences, and feedback" (1995, p. 66). Senge states, "From the system perspective, the human actor is the part of the feedback process, not standing apart from it. This is a profound shift in awareness" (1990, p. 78). The same can be said for simulation.

The human performance system framework provides a powerful mental model for diagnosing and addressing the root causes of deficient human performance. The SOS professional can use this framework when helping healthcare educators, performance improvement trainers, performance (competence) assessors, and researchers to design and evaluate simulation events to improve and/or assess performance. It supports the *purpose, practices,* and *partnership* elements of the 3×3 roles of simulation operations (see Fig. 7.3).

CONCLUSION

Healthcare simulation is standing in the foyer of amazing possibilities to improve and sustain the performance of the emerging and current healthcare professionals to provide patients and families with safe, quality healthcare. As technologies and caregiver disciplines become more complex and integrated, the role of the various simulation specialties must adapt to remain relevant. There will always be a need for simulation technicians who work their magic to make the simulation technologies function. Fulfilling the nine roles of simulation operations in the future will depend upon a profession that can bridge the gap between what simulation operations can offer to healthcare providers and educators to achieve valued performance accomplishments and results. The SOS professional can step into that gap by taking a Human Performance Value Stream perspective, integrating the nine roles of simulation operations, and providing a human performance system framework to help educators and clinicians diagnose and treat organizational barriers to performance, as well as human performance deficiencies. Perhaps, these three conceptual frameworks will also provide a different perspective during the technician/clinician/educator debate by providing a glimpse into future possibilities for this emerging profession.

REFERENCES

Addison, R., Haig, C., & Kearney, L. (2009). *Performance architecture: The art and science of improving organizations.* San Francisco: Pfeiffer.

Arnold, J. (2012, June 21). *Simulation for pediatric healthcare: Past, present, and future.* Paper presented at the The International Nursing Association for Clinical Simulation and Learning, San Antonio, TX.

Arthur, W., Bennett, W., Stanush, P. L., & McNelly, T. L. (1998). Factors that influence skills decay and retention: A quantitative review and analysis. *Human Performance, 11*(1), 57–101.

Binder, C. (2007). The six boxes: A descendent of gilbert's behavior engineering model. *Performance Improvement, 37*(6), 48–52.

Bond, S., & Cooper, S. (2006). Modelling emergency decisions: Recognition-primed decision making. The literature in relation to an opthalmic critical incident. *Journal of Clinical Nursing, 18*(8), 1023–1032.

Brethower, K. S. (1967). Maintenance systems: The neglected half of behavior change. In G. A. Rummler, J. P. Yaney, & A. W. Schrader (Eds.), *Managing the instructional programming effort* (pp. 60–72). An Arbor: Bureau of Industrial Relations, University of Michigan.

Brock, T. R. (2007, March). *Training nasa astronauts for deep space exploration missions: A research study to develop and validate a competency-based training framework.* Dissertation. (UMI No. 3255614). Ann Arbor, MI.

Buzachero, V. V., Phillips, J. J., Phillips, P. P., & Phillips, Z. L. (2013). *Measuring ROI in healthcare: Tools and techniques to measure the impact and ROI in healthcare improvement projects and programs.* New York: McGraw Hill Education.

Clark, R. C. (1999a). *Building expertise: Cognitive methods for training and performance improvement* (1st ed.). Washington, DC: International Society for Performance Improvement.

Clark, R. C. (1999b). *Developing technical training: A structured approach for developing classroom and computer-based instructional materials* (2nd ed.). Washington, DC: International Society for Performance Improvement.

Coleman, S. L., Menaker, E. S., & Murawski, M. (2000, November 27–30). *Maximizing technology integration efforts using a research-based approach.* Paper presented at the Interservice/Industry Training, Simulation, and Education Conference, Orlando, FL.

Dick, W., Carey, L., & Carey, J. O. (2014). *The systematic design of instruction* (8th ed.). New York: Longman.

Dylan, B. (1964). *The times they are a-changin'. On The Times They Are A-Changin'.* New York: Columbia Studios.

Foshay, W. R., Silber, K. H., & Stelnicki, M. (2003). *Writing training materials that work: How to train anyone to do anything.* San Francisco: Jossey-Bass/Pfeiffer.

Foster, T. C., Melon, E. G., & Phillips, H. L. (2007). Undergraduate military flight officer training: Increasing training effectiveness through job task and training media analysis. *Performance Improvement, 46*(3), 36–41.

Gagne, R. M., Briggs, L. J., & Wagner, W. M. (1992). *Principles of instructional design* (4th ed.). Belmont, CA: Wadsworth/Thornson Learning.

Gantt, L. (2012). Who's driving? The role and training of human patient simulation operator. *CIN: Computers, Informatics, Nursing, 30*(11), 579–586.

Gilbert, T. (1996). *Human competence: Engineering worthy performance.* Silver Spring, MD: International Society for Performance Improvement.

Gilbert, T. F., & Gilbert, M. B. (1989). Performance engineering: Making human productivity a science. *Performance and Instruction, 28*(1), 3–9.

Hale, J. (2012). *Performance-based evaluation: Tools and techniques to measure the impact of training.* San Francisco: Pfeiffer.

Handshaw, D. (2014). *Training that delivers results: Instructional design that aligns with business goals.* New York: AMACOM.

Harless, J. (1998). *The eden conspiracy: Educating for accomplished citizenships*. Wheaton, IL: Guild V Publications.

Hayden, J. K., Smiley, R. A., Alexander, M., Kardong-Edgren, S., & Jeffries, P. R. (2014). The NCSBN national simulation study: A longitudinal, randomized, controlled study replacing clinical hours with simulation in prelicensure nursing education. *Journal of Nursing Regulation, 5*(2), 66.

Hubbard, A., & Embrey, D. (2010). *Deepwater horizon—summary of critical events, human factors issues and implementations*. 10. Retrieved August 7, 2015 from http://humanreliability.com/documents/DeepwaterHorizon-HumanFactorsIssuesOG.pdf

Institute of Medicine. (1999). *To err is human: Building a safer healthcare system*. Washington, DC: National Academy Press.

Kaufman, R. (2000). *Mega planning: Practical tools for organizational success*. Thousand Oaks, CA: Sage Publications.

Kaufman, R., & Guerra-Lopez, I. (2013). *Needs assessment for organizational success*. Alexandria, VA: American Society for Training and Development.

Kaufman, R., Oakley-Brown, H., Watkins, R., & Lee, D. (2003). *Strategic planning for success: Aligning people, performance, and payoffs*. San Francisco: Jossey-Bass/Pfeiffer.

Kirkpatrick, D. L. (1994). *Evaluating training programs: The four levels*. San Francisco: Berrett-Koehler.

MacDonald, J., McDowell, P., Siegel, D., & DeLeon, J. R. (2014). Integrating games into learning environments. In T. S. Hussain & S. L. Coleman (Eds.), *Design and development of training games: Practical guidelines from a multidisciplinary perspective* (pp. 273–302). New York: Cambridge University Press.

Mager, R. F. (1997). *Preparing instructional objectives* (3rd ed.). Atlanta, GA: The Center for Effective Performance, Inc.

Mager, R. F., & Piper, P. (1997). *Analyzing performance problems* (3rd ed.). Atlanta, GA: The Center for Effective Performance, Inc.

Noe, R. A. (2013). *Employee training and development* (6th ed.). New York: McGraw-Hill Irwin.

Perrow, C. (1984). *Normal accidents: Living with high risk technologies*. Princeton: Princeton University Press.

Phillips, J. J. (1997). *Handbook of training evaluation and measurement methods* (3rd ed.). Houston, TX: Gulf Publishing Company.

Reason, J. (1997). *Managing the risks of organizational accidents*. Hampshire, UK: Ashgate Publishing Company.

Reason, J. (1999). *Human error*. Cambridge/New York: Cambridge University Press.

Rummler, G. A. (2004). *Serious performance consulting: According to Rummler*. Silver Springs, MD: International Society for Performance Improvement.

Rummler, G. A., & Brache, A. P. (1992). Transforming organizations through human performance technology. In H. D. Stolovitch & E. J. Keeps (Eds.), *Handbook of human performance technology: A comprehensive guide for analyzing and solving performance problems in organizations* (pp. 32–49). San Francisco: Jossey-Bass Publishers.

Rummler, G. A., & Brache, A. P. (1995). *Improving performance: How to manage the white space on the organizational chart*. San Francisco: Jossey-Bass.

Rush, R. M., Jr. (2013). Simulation in military and battlefield medicine. In A. Levine, S. DeMaria, Jr., A. Schwartz, & A. Sim (Eds.), *The comprehensive textbook of healthcare simulation* (pp. 401–413). New York: Springer.

Senge, P. M. (1990). *The fifth discipline: The art and practice of the learning organization.* New York: Currency Doubleday.

Skinner, A. (2014). *Retention and retraining of integrated cognitive and psychomotor skills.* Paper presented at the Interservice/Industry Training, Simulation, and Education Conference, Orlando, FL.

Society for Simulation in Healthcare. (2014). *About simulation.* Retrieved August 7, 2015 from http://www.ssih.org/About-Simulation

Swanson, R. A. (2007). *Analysis for improving performance: Tools for diagnosing organizations and documenting workplace expertise* (2nd ed.). San Francisco: Barrett-Koehler.

US Department of Defense. (2001). *Mil-hdbk-29612a, instructional systems development/systems approach to training and education (part 2 of 5 parts).* Washington, DC: US Government Printing Office.

US Department of Energy. (2009). *Doe-hdbk-1028-2009, human performance handbook: Vol. 1. Concepts and principles.* Washington, DC: US Government Printing Office.

8

FINDING THE FIT: WHAT THE SIMULATION OPERATIONS SPECIALIST HAS TO OFFER AND WHAT THE EMPLOYER NEEDS

AMAR PATEL

WakeMed Health & Hospitals, Raleigh, NC, USA

INTRODUCTION

Simulation has become an integral part of a wide variety of educational programs. The growing challenge for any program extends beyond understanding the role of simulation to the operations of the simulation space and its technology. Integration and operationalization of simulation technology is no easy tasks. The processes and methods involved and the technology itself all require a knowledgeable simulation operations specialist (SOS) with the ability to adapt to an evolving and unique environment.

There are two questions that must be asked within a simulation program. First, is a technology-savvy individual such as an SOS really needed to help create a nationally recognized simulation program? Lastly, when does such a person need to be added to the core team? Both are important questions that must be addressed early on by either simulation center management or the leadership team responsible for integrating simulation technology. Despite the financial debates that will surely arise about adding full-time employees to the team, an SOS is essential in ensuring that a program is successful in meeting its core mission, vision, and values. Without this particular team member, the technology may not be efficiently or effectively utilized.

Healthcare Simulation: A Guide for Operations Specialists, First Edition.
Edited by Laura T. Gantt and H. Michael Young.
© 2016 John Wiley & Sons, Inc. Published 2016 by John Wiley & Sons, Inc.

What is the best approach to acquiring an SOS for a program? For starters, an understanding of what healthcare employers are looking for in an SOS is required. This chapter will explore three diverse perspectives on the role of the SOS. The first is as a healthcare system, the second is as an emergency medical services (EMS) education program, and last is as an academic program. We focus on these particular areas because the needs, demands, as well as the mission, vision, and values, are unique in each of these environments; because of these, the job requirements for an SOS will also be different. With an understanding of what employers may be looking for, exploring what qualifications an SOS should have and how an SOS is essential in creating a simulation-based educational program becomes simpler.

THE EMPLOYER'S NEEDS

What a program needs versus what it wants can lead to two very different sets of pre-requisites in developing a job description and hiring a qualified individual. Many employers develop job descriptions based on the "perfect" candidate and create criteria for an individual that may never meet the true needs of the simulation center. Others create a job description based on an individual programmatic need. So, what is the perfect balance?

Regardless of the setting in which simulation-based education is being conducted, whether it is academic, EMS, or hospital, the core knowledge of the individual in this position must include a basic understanding of technology integration. The term technology integration could mean networking infrastructure, biomedical engineering, computer programming, or even audio-visual installation and design, to name a few. In the end, the SOS must be able to understand the technical components of the simulation hardware and software, and be able to incorporate that into any new or existing infrastructure. The true test of a technologically savvy individual is their ability to take an unknown piece of technology and, with a little bit of time, understand it and integrate it into any system.

The Healthcare System

A few case examples may prove helpful. Jane is the Chief Nursing Officer at Mills Health Care. She has experience in establishing a simulation program, but is not familiar with how an SOS may contribute to an already functional simulation center. Jane's simulation educator, Marcy, is her only simulation education specialist (SES); Marcy recently completed her Certified Healthcare Simulation Educator (CHSE) certification through the Society for Simulation in Healthcare (SSH). As part of her certification preparation, Marcy learned about the importance of an SOS and the role an SOS plays in the day-to-day operations of a simulation center.

Marcy is the sole educator in the nursing education department responsible for delivering simulation-based education; she is often tasked with developing and delivering the education, and with troubleshooting the technology also. On occasion, Marcy is able to solicit the help of the biomedical engineering and information technology departments.

However, both of these departments are already overwhelmed with normal operations; each unit often expresses concern about their familiarity with the technology and the process to integrate the simulation and audio-visual systems in the current network infrastructure. After carefully reviewing the requirements outlined by the SSH for a Certified Healthcare Simulation Operations Specialist (CHSOS), Marcy proposes that Mills Health Care hire an SOS who meets many of the criteria as established by SSH for the newly created position. Jane expresses her concerns with hiring an additional full-time person (full-time equivalent or FTE) and wants a detailed job description that would support adding an SOS to the existing simulation program. Marcy is asked to highlight key job requirements that help meet the basic needs of the health-care system, while also outlining those additional needs to be met by the SOS that would take the Mills Health Care simulation program to the next level.

After review of the CHSOS requirements and discussion of the role of an SOS with the hospital's biomedical engineering and information technology departments, Marcy reaches out to similar hospital-based simulation programs in her country. She learns that the role of an SOS is relatively new, but that there is a clear need to have a technology-savvy individual who can facilitate the day-to-day simulation operations. For hospital-based programs, Marcy learns that the SOS must have a Bachelor's degree in a healthcare field with experience in education delivery, information technology, and simulation technology. Marcy also learns that, while there are similarities between informational technology and simulation technology, the differences in the technology and the level of diversity across disciplines is what separates the two. She finds that the SOS must understand education, simulation, and healthcare to be effective in the role of an SOS, whereas traditional informational technology or biomedical engineers are technology-specific experts. The diversity of experience is what makes the role of the SOS so unique in simulation and healthcare.

Marcy expresses to Jane her desire to have an individual with a Bachelor's degree that has strong critical thinking skills and healthcare experience with a preference for a person in healthcare simulation education. Jane added that her desire would be to have an SOS with a minimum of two years of experience in simulation. Jane's preference for 2 years of experience matches the SSH requirement for a CHSOS, which is based on an understanding of the amount of time it takes an individual to develop a strong foundational knowledge of simulation operations. She discusses the need for a person who is flexible and has diverse understanding of simulation, audio-visual, information technology, technological hardware design and troubleshooting, and basic software programming. Furthermore, the preferred SOS candidate must be detail oriented with strong time management skills.

What Marcy found was that Mills Health Care really did not know what the job description of an SOS should be. Mills Health Care has a basic understanding of what makes an SOS an important part of a simulation program, but is still learning how to best utilize the SOS in the simulation center. Their end goal was for the program to have an experienced individual that could immediately make an impact on patient outcomes and provider safety, while making substantive contributions to the growth of innovation throughout the system. An educator dedicated to simulation-based education could accomplish all of these goals, but without an individual with technical and operational knowledge of simulation, immediate impact would be more difficult to achieve.

It is easy to forget that the simulation center is a business with customers and a mandate to provide a clear return on investment (ROI) for their organization. This requires a strong and knowledgeable team of individuals that believe in making an impact and clearly do that. Marcy and Jane agreed that the SOS is an important member of that team. Both believe they have a strong job description with clear gaps identified in their current healthcare system to be able to show how an SOS would be utilized; the role would also potentially decrease the overall demands of the simulation center on informational technology and biomedical engineering.

Emergency Medical Services

Jim is the director of education for ABS Ambulance Service. He recently learned about simulation at a conference and became interested in expanding ABS Ambulance Service's educational programs to include the utilization of human patient simulators. Jim has the funding he needs to add a full-time SOS, but is not sure what the qualifications of this new employee should be. He knows that an SOS should be a credentialed EMS provider in the event that this individual needs to respond to an emergency. Jim and his education program team members are familiar with simulation, since much of EMS education utilizes many of the fundamental principles highlighted by simulation educators, including prebriefings, scripted scenario development, a simulation experience, and debriefings. However, the integration of high-fidelity simulation technology, use of audio-visual systems for recording simulation experiences, and the scheduling of equipment are all new to Jim. In hopes of finding a "jack of all trades," Jim begins to work on putting together the perfect job description for an SOS.

Jim takes the time to reach out to other EMS organizations around the country that utilize human patient simulators. He learns that some programs do not have an SOS simply because of budget constraints and therefore rotate staff through their training academy. This results in individuals having a mixed level of experience with high fidelity training equipment and inconsistency in the delivery of training across the EMS agency. Jim hopes to avoid incidences of uneven education delivery by utilizing a dedicated SOS. The dedicated SOS, in conjunction with core educators that can be routinely rotated through the training academy, will allow for consistent use of the simulation technology. Furthermore, this will allow educators to teach those topic areas with which they are most comfortable.

After careful review of the CHSOS requirements and the information provided by other EMS organizations, Jim determines that the perfect SOS should be a seasoned EMS provider with experience or familiarity in EMS education. Although the CHSOS application highlights the need for an individual to have a Bachelor's degree, it also provides an avenue for those that do not to show how their education and professional experience would be equal to the degree itself. Jim realizes the challenges in finding an experienced EMS professional with a Bachelor's degree. He further understands the value in such a degree since it demonstrates acquisition of knowledge in key areas, such as the basic sciences, English, and even time management skills.

However, the requirement for a Bachelor's degree is negotiable for Jim if the individual is able to prove experience is commensurate to the degree itself. Jim believes that, in addition to being an EMS provider, the SOS should have strong time management skills, be flexible, have the ability to manage multiple projects at the same time, and have an expert level of knowledge of technology. Jim believes that for ABS Ambulance Service, the SOS should be able to integrate and troubleshoot simulation technology, audio-visual systems, and helps ensure that education is consistently delivered. Jim's choice to have someone who can perform a variety of job duties is key to ensuring that the funding available for the full-time employee equivalent is fully justified. Furthermore, having an experienced SOS work with an EMS education expert will help ABS Ambulance Service improve use of simulation methodology across the service and challenge any generation of EMS professionals.

Academia

As Jane, Marcy, and Jim had opportunities to speak with their respective counterparts at local university simulation programs and community colleges, they learned that both programs provided education to nursing students and allied healthcare professionals, such as EMS and dentistry. The university simulation program also provided education to the pharmacy school, the anesthesia program, the medical school, and the physical therapy program. They all expressed the importance of having a strong group of simulation educators, technologists, and operations specialists. Although the desire for a dedicated simulation technologist is important, the role of the SOS can be multifaceted enough to allow them to be a technologist for many aspects of the day-to-day operations of a small to medium size simulation program. In the academic environment, where a simulation center may conduct several thousand simulations per year, it is important for both the simulation technologist and the SOS to be active members of the simulation program. For those programs that are new to simulation or just beginning to utilize simulation-based education principles in their curriculum, an SOS and a simulation educator will provide that program with the appropriate level of structure and guidance. The integration of a simulation technologist is only necessary when the types of equipment and the amount of equipment varies enough that a technologist is required to redesign or reconfigure the space and the equipment on a routine basis. The true role of an SOS is to provide guidance and support in the day-to-day operations, in addition to managing the technological needs of the simulation program.

Like her counterparts Jane, Marcy, and Jim, Kelly recently took over as the operations director for CDS University's Center for Innovation and Learning (Fig. 8.1). CDS is new to high-fidelity simulation. They first encountered this technology with an in situ simulation last year after receiving funds for a low-fidelity training manikin. CDS was able to utilize this portable technology in their own facility with minimal support from the manufacturer and limited education. The technology controlling the manikin was intuitive enough that an educator was able to run simulations alone without much difficulty. However, as the complexity of the technology has grown in recent years and as numerous CDS educators have voiced the desire to

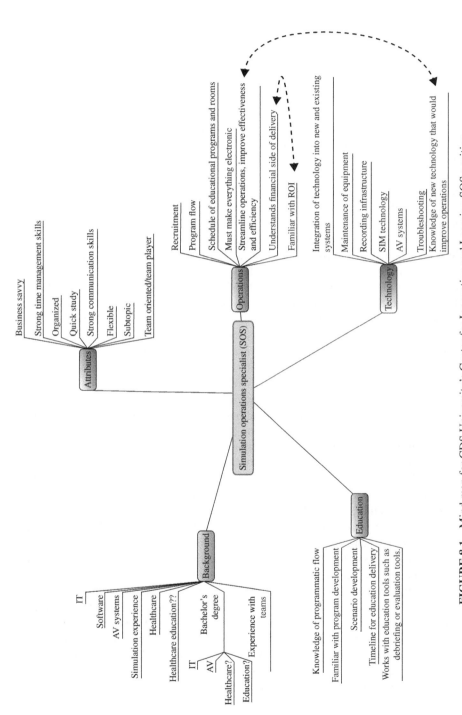

FIGURE 8.1 Mind map for CDS University's Center for Innovation and Learning SOS position.

increase the fidelity of simulation experiences, Kelly has begun to explore adding on an SOS to her center's staff. She believes that the SOS can be vital in helping the educators standardize the process by which simulation is delivered. Furthermore, she hopes that the SOS will be able to help program patient care scenarios using any simulation technology platform in order to meet programmatic needs and ensure consistency in student experiences.

Kelly begins by outlining what the organization hopes the SOS will be able to accomplish upon joining the team. She begins by utilizing mind mapping software to help her piece together all of the different jobs that the SOS would have (Appendix 2). The software helped Kelly visually organize all of the information currently available about an SOS and the organization's wishes for that role. The unique structure of a mind map is able to help Kelly add or delete various components of the SOS job so that she can better understand how complex the job can be. Her mind map reveals a large number of responsibilities for an individual that must demonstrate expertise in technology, time management, and program operations. Kelly further finds that the SOS must be able to think quickly and critically, and adapt to ongoing modifications in a fluid simulation environment, an ever-changing array of technology, and a constantly evolving set of academic requirements. In addition to this unique set of skills, Kelly feels that the SOS must have some connection to or knowledge about healthcare. Although she feels strongly that the individual needs to be a healthcare professional by certification or licensure, the ideal SOS candidate should also have completed courses that would provide a basic understanding of medical terminology, anatomy, physiology, and pathophysiology. With the direct connection the SOS would have to clinical professionals and the need to program and run their scenarios, the SOS must also understand the case structure in order to translate that information in to a simulation experience. Similar to the hospital-based or EMS setting, the SOS would not be making decisions on the structure or content of the educational program, but rather translating what has been designed into the simulation technology.

With a long list of job-related duties determined and the need for the SOS to be flexible based on the needs of the program, the last consideration Kelly must make relates to is educational requirements. Should the SOS have an undergraduate degree or something more? After careful review of a pay scale range for an SOS, CDS's human resource department recommended that candidates for the position should have a Bachelor's degree in an information technology or healthcare field. Although a professional certification shows validity and expertise in a given field, the Bachelor's degree shows achievements in basic skills that are needed to be successful in an academic environment. For some time, Kelly debated the needed for the SOS to have a graduate degree matching those of many of her staff members and educators in the Center for Innovation and Learning. However, she also considered the possibility that the graduate degree would not provide any additional value in the newly developed SOS role. After all, this individual would need to have strong technical and operational knowledge, something that is achieved with a combination of hands-on experience and technical education. Kelly believed that the Bachelor's degree requirement, as matches the CHSOS certification, would be sufficient.

In the academic setting, the institution may require the SOS to complete additional certifications and education to ensure that they are able to meet the needs of the department. The growing challenge in this environment is the constantly evolving list of requirements for both the students and the faculty. Although the SOS would not have any direct teaching role, they would be interacting with students and indirectly impacting how they process new knowledge and skills. In this particular setting, the SOS must help the simulation educator creating a safe, confidential, and unique learning environment where learners are able to immediately apply new knowledge. If the SOS fails to help create that environment, then the student could fail to understand the value of that content. The role of the SOS is important in ensuring the student receives any and all methods of learning that may be possible within the simulation program. Kelly recognizes that the SOS may be the backbone in the simulation program's success.

KNOWLEDGE OF SIMULATION

Simulation is an educational methodology. The focus of simulation is to create an environment where students are safe to make mistakes. In these environments, students learn from their mistakes and that lesson helps them understand the relevance and impact a mistake can make to a patient. In the end, these lessons improve both patient and provider safety. They also help improve the quality of care being delivered across the entire healthcare spectrum. The knowledge an SOS must possess includes understanding how valuable simulation is. The role of the operations specialists is to create a realistic enough environment that the student's level of interaction increases as the simulation scenario progresses. An SOS sets the stage for what the SES and the student hope will be an amazing simulation experience. A successful education experience is evident early on in the simulation as the SES begins to see critical thinking skills being utilized and the predetermined objectives being met. For an SOS to be effective, he/she must be able to help educators obtain any relevant data needed for research studies or assist educators in replaying valuable video for debriefings. An SOS and simulation educator work hand-in-hand in delivering a high-quality educational program or conducting a valuable research study. The knowledge the SOS possesses is valuable to the simulation program.

THEMES

A careful look at how Mills Health Care, ABS Ambulance Service, and CDS University's Center for Innovation and Learning approached adding an SOS position revealed several themes about the position itself. Furthermore, their approaches to developing a job description and seeking approval for the full-time employee highlights the need for any program to research how the SOS would be used within the simulation center. In all, six themes emerged from the research conducted by all three educational programs.

Undergraduate Degree

The Bachelor's degree demonstrates that the SOS is able to understand simple and complex thought. With this degree, the SOS has developed critical thinking skills, enhanced their communication skills, developed time management skills, and mastered the ability to carry out thoughtful reflection with others. Although the requirement for a Bachelor's degree can be debated depending on where the SOS may be working, the skills obtained while completing a Bachelor's degree are difficult to substitute with professional experience. However, in the right professional atmosphere, an SOS may be able to learn key strategies and skills that could prove to be just as valuable as those obtained while completing an undergraduate degree. In addition to the developing a wide variety of core skills while in college, the ability for the student to be exposed to various technical and social environments further enhances diversity. Students, while in school, are exposed to a wide variety of ethnicities and cultures, and they are forced to communicate with others in a meaningful way that teaches them how both positive and negative interactions should occur. Although life experiences may provide some of this exposure, the diversity of individuals and groups across a college campus may opt be duplicated elsewhere. As the role of the SOS evolves, the Bachelor's degree requirement is likely to become non-negotiable.

Certifications and Licensures

Jim from ABS Ambulance Service revealed early on that any individual assigned to provide EMS education must be an experienced and credentialed EMS provider or be able to obtain the necessary EMS certification. Jim's rationale for requiring an EMS certification was twofold. First, Jim felt that the SOS must be knowledgeable about the environment in which and how EMS education is conducted as well as the language used. The only way to accomplish this is by having direct experience in EMS. Second, the SOS must be able to provide emergency medical care if called upon. Although Jim's preference is for a currently certified EMS provider with pre-hospital care experience, he realizes that he may have to train someone. The requirement for a technical or professional certification or licensure will be dependent on where the SOS is assigned. While an EMS agency may require an EMS certification, an academic or healthcare environment may require the SOS to have some type of professional computer certification such as CompTIA A+, Microsoft Certified Professional, or Certified Technology Specialist (CTS). How the SOS will be utilized in the simulation center, where the SOS will be assigned to work, and any additional duties the SOS may be required to perform will dictate what professional certifications must be obtained. The role of the SOS as defined by all three programs described in this chapter clearly indicates that a professional healthcare licensure, such as a nursing license, would not be required. Although there is value in having that additional awareness while performing in the SOS role, the knowledge obtained by completing a nursing degree may be better utilized by for those wishing to become simulation educators.

Knowledgeable in Instructional Systems Design

To be a valuable member of the simulation team, the SOS should have some foundational knowledge in educational principles and instructional system design theory. Although an SOS's role is operational in nature, he or she helps the simulation educator connect all of the various operational needs for successful simulation experiences. By having an understanding of instructional theories, the SOS can ensure that the content placed into an operational format has an identified problem statement, a completed needs assessment, clear goals and objectives, an implementation process, and an evaluation (Cook et al., 2013; Robinson & Dearmon, 2013).

In addition to understanding instructional system design, the SOS should have a solid grasp on the principles of debriefing and feedback. While the SOS works to manage the technology and interpret the developed simulation experience, an understanding of how the feedback and debriefing will be conducted aids in seeing the entire process through to completion. As an operations specialist, the SOS provides feedback on the session, recommendations on how to improve the experience, and confirms that the delivered content matches the original instructional design plan. To ensure the simulation experience meets the specified training need, the SOS should assist with creating supplemental materials such as checklists. An important aspect of any instructional design is vetting and testing the simulation experience. The SOS must work with the simulation educator and other content experts to pilot the simulation experience and ensure it has been flawlessly designed. At the conclusion of testing process, the SOS should assist the simulation educator in developing assessment tools that match the operational needs of the simulation program and the organization. Lastly, once the supplemental materials have been created and the scenario has been piloted, the SOS must collaborate with content experts in designing and deploying the debriefing. The SOS's knowledge of the simulation center's operations helps with development of additional courses and organizational processes that may add value to students seeking additional simulation experiences.

Team Functionality is Crucial

Teamwork involves working with fellow peers, customers, and leadership in developing a simulation experience and simulation center that can drive improvements in healthcare. While much of the SOS's role is to understand the components of simulation operations, learning theory, and simulation technology, it is equally important for the SOS to be a strong team player. Knowing how the SOS will work with others is important in gauging impact on the team environment. Some simple questions to ask yourself as the employer or as a future SOS are as follows:

- Does the prospective SOS work well with other team members or prefer to work independently?
- Does the SOS understand the role of each member in the simulation center?
- Does the SOS understand how to work collaboratively with others?
- Is the SOS willing to admit being wrong or allow others to win arguments?

- Has the SOS historically worked in a team environment?
- Does the SOS feel like he/she can delegate tasks or prefer to complete everything?
- Is the SOS a teacher or advocate for simulation-based education?
- Is the SOS an attentive listener?

Each of these questions may help the future SOS understand how they interact with their environment. It can also be valuable to know where the SOS and the team are on Myers-Briggs Type Indicators (Allchin, Dzurec, & Engler, 2009). This simple personality inventory can help the employee and employer understand how team members will interact with each other. Although it cannot be used as part of the hiring decision, it can be a valuable tool in understanding how effective the team will be.

Multi-Tasking and Time Management

Multi-tasking and time management require someone who clearly understands how to navigate checklists and calendars well. The growing challenge with multi-tasking is that the individual must understand personal limitations. Simply put, multi-tasking is all about managing multiple tasks, yet what many fail to realize is that in the process of juggling tasks, only so much concentration can be devoted to any one task. For example, let us speculate that the SOS was attempting to type a summary on the operational process for integrating a pediatric scenario in to a pediatric residency program while the simulation educator is asking for assistance in getting another simulation experience scheduled before the end of the business day. Is the SOS able to complete the summary and coordinate getting the simulation experience scheduled? What takes priority? Even though Mills Health Care, ABS Ambulance Service, and the Center for Innovation and Learning all specified the need for an SOS that can multi-task, the employer should ask themselves how effective can a multi-tasker be? Instead of being able to multi-task, the SOS should have strong time management skills and understand how to prioritize various tasks. By strengthening time management skills, the SOS will be able to meet the needs of their employers and the busy simulation program. A highly impactful program is only as good as the individual team members that can manage various assigned responsibilities and not attempt to do all the tasks at the same time.

Diversity of Experience

The amount of personal and professional experience an SOS brings to the simulation center may determine how effective the simulation operations will be. Early on, all three of the healthcare educational programs discussed in this chapter identified the need for an SOS with a diverse background in education, healthcare, and technology. So what does that diversity need to include? How diverse is not diverse enough?

The individual simulation programs must determine the amount and type of diversity they need. While some program may choose to have a technology-savvy individual with strong time management skills who is a licensed practitioner with educational experience, others may simply need a technology-savvy individual. The ever-changing simulation environment makes knowing how to define diversity a bit more difficult. However, it is safe to surmise that an SOS should have a strong foundational knowledge in technology and education, and, when possible, healthcare education. For programs like the ABS Ambulance Service, the requirement may also include pre-hospital emergency care or education experience. The unique nature of simulation and the various roles an SOS may play makes developing an exact job description challenging. Nevertheless, the primary role of the SOS is to facilitate the operations of the simulation environment; by developing a strong technical understanding of the technology, the SOS can be a valuable member of the team.

All members of the simulation teams offer a variety of skills and it is not uncommon for the simulation educator to have as strong an operational understanding as the SOS. After all, the simulation educator is tasked with developing the education that the students will actually use in taking care of patients. The term *diversity* is utilized to help the employer and the prospective SOS recognize that any new employee will need to have knowledge in multiple areas when it comes to simulation. One day the SOS may be running scenarios in the hospital environment, while the next day that same SOS is working in a simulated active shooter environment. The world around healthcare is constantly changing. It is up to the SOS to help others understand how creative simulation can be. The more experience and exposure the SOS has had, the more they can do with the simulation team.

CONCLUSION

As illustrated by the three case examples outlined in this chapter, the need for an SOS in any simulation program is clear. However, what is often debated is how to justify funding the SOS position long term. Future SOSs must sell themselves as individuals who may easily adapt to the changing healthcare and simulation market. A strong applicant for an SOS position should be able to speak to the value of the role in a simulation program and demonstrate how the knowledge brought will demonstrate a ROI to the organization. For organizations that are interested in hiring an SOS but unsure of where to begin, reaching out to others and asking for help is the best route. The role of an SOS is unique and one that will help any simulation program excel. It is important to know what is needed, how an SOS is going to be utilized, and what the requirements for that role need to be within that organization. In the end, the SOS can be your most innovative person, driving the growth of the simulation program while building relationships between disciplines.

REFERENCES

Allchin, L., Dzurec, L. C., & Engler, A. J. (2009). Psychological type and explanatory style of nursing students and clinical faculty. *Journal of Nursing Education, 48*(4), 196–202.

Cook, D. A., Hamstra, S. J., Brydges, R., Zendejas, B., Szostek, J. H., Wang, A. T., Hatala, R. (2013). Comparative effectiveness of instructional design features in simulation-based education: Systematic review and meta-analysis. *Medical Teacher, 35*, e867–e898. doi:10.3109/0142159X.2012.714886

Robinson, B. K., & Dearmon, V. (2013). Evidence-Based nursing education: Effective use of instructional design and simulated learning environments to enhance knowledge transfer in undergraduate nursing students. *Journal of Professional Nursing, 29*(4), 203–209. doi:10.1016/j.profnurs.2012.04.022

9

FOUNDATIONS FOR THE SIMULATION OPERATIONS SPECIALIST

EVAN J. BARTLEY

ECU College of Nursing, Greenville, NC, USA

INTRODUCTION

When considering the desired skillset of the simulation operations specialist (SOS), the primary question that needs to be asked is, "what is expected of someone who assumes this new role?" Since the use of simulation in healthcare education is relatively new, the possibility exists that the person hired to fill a role within simulation operations would have previous experience in any of several roles related to that of the SOS. In an effort to help prepare newly hired SOSs who are expected to perform duties related to healthcare simulation operations, this chapter discusses the development of an orientation process, or guide, to address skillsets and processes that are typically expected of an SOS.

Categorizing the skills into *fields* or *domains* necessitates a clear understanding of the simulation center's overall mission and how the expected skills affect the scope of the SOS's position.

In 2015, the Society for Simulation in Healthcare's (SSH) Committee for Certification completed the pilot phase of the *Certified Healthcare Simulation Operations Specialist* (CHSOS) professional certification program and announced its first recipients of the coveted and highly anticipated credential. The process for developing this kind of certification includes a rigorous job analysis of the roles and skillsets within operations that included exemplars from other industries, in addition

Healthcare Simulation: A Guide for Operations Specialists, First Edition.
Edited by Laura T. Gantt and H. Michael Young.
© 2016 John Wiley & Sons, Inc. Published 2016 by John Wiley & Sons, Inc.

to healthcare, where both simulation and operations were both key elements. The *SSH Certified Healthcare Simulation Operations Specialist Handbook* outlines the process and nature of the exam, the knowledge, skills, and abilities required of an CHSOS, as well as the expectations of that process. Within this handbook is an outline of the five major domains and elements within each domain that provide a "blueprint" for the examination content. The *blueprint* informs the candidate about the content domains of the CHSOS exam. This chapter is informed by the CHSOS examination blueprint, but does not address *all* elements of the blueprint.

SOS RECRUITMENT AND ONBOARDING

How does management orient the SOS to a program? The responsibilities, skills, and expectations of an SOS may be categorized into five different *fields* (domains). The identification of these fields should serve two purposes:

1. To analyze the candidate's experience against defined knowledge, skills, and attributes;
2. To identify those areas of experience lacking in a candidate, and determine what training, if any, will be required.

First, evaluating a candidate's experience to see if their previous job tasks and responsibilities align with any of the fields mentioned in this chapter, and the CHSOS handbook, will assist decision-makers in identifying the most desirable applicants. Categorizing an applicant's responsibilities by professional background or experience allows one to identify common skills that are useful to an SOS. The SOS would also benefit from a self-evaluation of personal and professional skills as they relate to expectations defined for this type of position. For example, a paramedic of 5 years will have expansive knowledge of pre-hospital healthcare practice. However, this paramedic should also examine the skills in the field of healthcare that typically pertain to the role and discover elements that may or may not have existed inside the paramedic's purview. This paramedic will likely possess an extensive range of skills that may not be expected of the typical SOS. There may also be some additional skills or procedures from the healthcare field that the paramedic may need to learn or review. This chapter will explore reasonable expectations of the SOS role.

Secondly, the content pertaining to a field in which one has little or no experience will help determine the types of training that should be pursued in order to prepare for service as an SOS. A person who is new to the role of the SOS will be unlikely to have all of the experience required to address the elements of the five fields, which are as follows:

1. SOS Foundations from the World of Information Technology
2. SOS Foundations from the World of Audiovisual Technology
3. SOS Foundations from the World of Theater and Drama
4. SOS Foundations from the World of Academia
5. SOS Foundations from the World of Healthcare

Each of the sections seeks not only to describe the skills and expectations that are associated with a particular field of study, but also to correlate those skills to the environment of simulation in healthcare education. Even those with extensive experience in one of the five fields of study would be prudent to investigate how skills from each field relate to the world of healthcare simulation. These categories also help provide a framework in which those seeking to hire an SOS could generate an orientation to the skills expected of such an individual. This is meant to provide a framework; skills from particular fields could go beyond the scope of an SOS at any given institution.

SOS FOUNDATIONS FROM THE WORLD OF INFORMATION TECHNOLOGY

The field of Information Technology (IT) (also known as: *information systems*) is a broad and ever-evolving landscape of new technologies and standards. From the advances of cloud storage and browser-based applications to biometric security features, IT is a field that offers innovation and adaptation as an answer to questions generated from all aspects of our world; healthcare simulation is no exception. An SOS will find that the field of IT plays a primary role in bringing a simulated environment to more and more healthcare education centers. The IT concepts discussed in this section serve as an incomplete list, but will address the common competencies and skills expected of an SOS.

Computer Hardware

Hardware refers to those parts of a computer that are *tangible*. They can be seen, handled, and take up physical space in the "real" world. The SOS should be able to *identify* the basic hardware components of a personal computer that include the following:

- Motherboard (system board),
- Graphics or video card (sometimes referred to as the Graphic Processing Unit (GPU)),
- Central processing unit (CPU),
- Random access memory (RAM),
- Expansion slots (PCI, PCI-Express, SAS, etc.),
- Universal serial bus (USB) ports,
- Ethernet card, port, network interface card (NIC),
- WiFi or wireless network card,
- Disc drives (CD, DVD, BluRay),
- Hard disk drive (HDD), aka the disk drive
- Monitor, screen, display.

The presence of various computer hardware components is clearly evident in many devices used in the simulated environment. Many of these components are also contained in commonly used manikin-based patient simulators. Several manufacturers of simulators seek to emulate human physiology and characteristics using computer hardware components. One popular manikin houses a complete computer, including motherboard (or system board), central processing unit (CPU or processor), Ethernet connection (such as network interface card or NIC), and other components.

The SOS should be familiar with the different types of computer video output and input ports as well. One potential complication of standard PC monitor configurations is the use of non-standard *drivers* to interface with a touchscreen monitor or touchscreen all-in-one computer for interfacing touch control with proprietary control software. *Drivers* are a type of software designed to "tell" a computer how to communicate with a physical device; more information on drivers is found in the next section pertaining to *software*. Simulation spaces may utilize both digital and analog computer video connections, where the control computer utilizes a digital connection (such as a DVI-D interface) for the primary monitor and at the same time using an extended desktop analog connection for the patient vital sign monitor (VGA). Information on the differences between digital and analog video is discussed in upcoming sections conjunction with information on common video connections.

Computer Software

The SOS will likely have direct interaction with computer software, either as an operator or provider of computer desktop support and maintenance. *Software* refers to the intangible components of computer systems. *Software* is often thought of as floppy disks, CDs, and flash drives. However, these devices are actually *hardware* (Andrews, 2013). You can see and touch a flash drive, for example. The software is actually stored on such devices. Software cannot be seen or touched in the real world, but can be manipulated through other software tools. Software can be generally classified as follows:

- Operating System or *OS*, such as:
  ◦ Microsoft Windows™
  ◦ Apple MacOS™
  ◦ Linux™
- Firmware
  ◦ BIOS (Basic Input Output System); software instructions that define how the system board interfaces with the various components that are interconnected on the system board, including ports, GPU, CPU, and RAM.
  ◦ Some might argue that the BIOS should be classified as hardware, but again, the hardware is only the medium by which the BIOS is stored and accessed.
- Drivers
  ◦ Specific software instructions that bridge the operating system with the hardware on the system board or devices connected to the various external ports available on a computer.

- Applications, such as:
  - Microsoft Office™ (and other productivity suites)
  - Google Chrome™ (and other browsers)
  - Manufacturer specific simulation control software
- File
  - A *file* is that part of the software that is generated when a user saves a document, image or script.
  - A program can be composed of hundreds of individual files, or can be as simple as one file that scripts computer behaviors.

Many simulation technologies can utilize various types of files that are common on many general office computers. For example, a Portable Document Format (PDF) file and other file types, including image files (pictures) are examples of file types that could be made available to scenario participants by an SOS. Such files can be exhibited as lab results, X-ray images, patient documentation, and pretty much any other type of file needed for the objectives of the scenario. An SOS will need to be familiar with most common file types used in a typical office setting. A list of common file types and related programs can be found in Appendix 4. It is worth noting that some computers, regardless of operating system, may not be configured to display the file type extensions. Enabling this feature would be helpful to an SOS but may need to be configured by the IT department depending on the computer's configuration. "Extensions" in this context refer to the file name type descriptor including a perod (.) and several characters. For example the extension of a PDF file is actually ".pdf" and a Microsoft Word file is ".docx".

SERIOUS GAMES

With the increased popularity of serious gaming applications that allow the learning context to exist in a computer gaming environment or virtual environment also comes additional complexity. Advancement in computer gaming has made it possible to train learners on the procedures found in and outside of clinical environments as well as practical skills found in healthcare. This creates a challenge for the SOS when such programs require specific computer specifications such as an OS version, additional RAM, or specialized graphic card upgrades.

MULTIPLE PLATFORM EXPERIENCE

Experience with more than one simulator platform is useful since many simulation programs utilize various brands and models. An SOS would be disadvantaged with experience in only one manufacturer's simulator. While there are similarities between proprietary systems, manikins may interface with control computers in different ways; the layout of the control software itself may also differ. For example, Laerdal Medical's products traditionally operate with a Microsoft Windows operating system, while CAE Healthcare simulators have Apple MacOS systems, although some of CAE's simulator control software can be run using a browser on a Windows computer. Variations in operating systems become obvious in working with different manufacturers of simulation-related products and are also increasingly evident as end users begin switching between personal computers and mobile devices. An SOS will find that technology support responsibilities necessitate familiarization with these varied platforms when working with learners, faculty, and colleagues.

An SOS should be able to distinguish between software products. As mentioned, the platform, or operating system, used by a computer enables the machine to run applications. Many applications are developed for multiple platforms, enabling files to be opened on different platforms. Microsoft, for example, designs *Microsoft Word*™ (a word processor) for both Windows™ and Macintosh™ platforms. There are many applications that only run on a single type of operating system. *Final Cut*® would be an example of a video editing application that is designed for an Apple Macintosh™ and cannot be used on a Windows machine.

DRIVERS

Another type of software encountered by operations specialists, as mentioned previously, is a *driver*. *Driver software* is a type of code, stored as a file, that enables an operating system to communicate with a device or hardware component. A common example is a driver that enables a computer system to utilize the unique capabilities of a video or graphics card. This software acts as a set of instructions by which the operating system (e.g. Windows™) and applications can utilize the graphics card. This type of software, or code, is not typically altered or summoned manually by the user but is utilized by operating systems every time the system is started. As long as a driver works correctly, little support is required. However, there are automatic updates to operating systems and hardware that require the driver to also be updated for it to function in the new environment. Manufacturers may also implement stability, security, or performance improvements and issue updates to driver software. Many times, responsibility falls to the SOS to manage and perform driver updates when the IT department is overwhelmed with other activities. Device failures during simulation sessions necessitates that the SOS initiates a troubleshooting process that may include reinstalling the driver or reverting to an older version of the software.

UTILITIES

Another type of software that an SOS will encounter is a *utility*. *Utility software* is designed to enhance or repair the operating system. In some cases, utilities are small programs meant to improve user productivity. Common types of computer system utilities include anti-virus or malware, disk defragmenter, file synchronization, and registry cleanup. This type of software is similar to an application in functionality, but is designed to be a tool to manage aspects of the computer. An example of a utility that is commonly utilized in the simulation environment is a network utility. This is a tool that alters the network configuration settings of a computer and manages the network connection so that applications work properly.

COMPUTER NETWORKS

In current simulation environments, the SOS relies on both wired and wireless communication. Some patient simulators are controlled over the local area network (LAN) (wired) or the wireless network (WiFi). A network is also used to control some *Pan-Tilt-Zoom* (PTZ) cameras. The SOS must be able to identify and describe the function of the components of a LAN. Common networking devices found in healthcare simulation include routers, switches, network interface cards (NICs), firewalls, wireless access points (WAP), and various connectors and cables. Refer to Appendix 3 for help identifying common connectors and related uses found in the simulation environment.

WIRED VERSUS WIRELESS NETWORKS

In addition to WiFi and Ethernet network communications, a less common network medium utilizes radio frequency (RF). Gaumard Scientific™ produces patient simulators that are not WiFi enabled, but rather uses RF for simulator control. An important aspect of RF to consider is that WiFi can interfere with signal strength (and vice versa). WiFi (IEEE 802.11b,g,n) and RF (IEEE 802.15) will both fight for the same space and many times use the same frequency (i.e. 2.4 GHz). Bluetooth (IEEE 802.15.1) also uses 2.4 GHz and would have to fight for the same space as RF and WiFi. Even though these devices operate and compete for the same air space, it is possible to have reliable operation with multiple devices in the same area. Typically, testing the environment with all of the devices to be used is the most helpful way to determine whether there is a problem. If communication slows or stops with wireless LAN and RF devices that typically operate well independently, physically rearranging the devices might help alleviate the problem. Some simulation centers have banned the use of cell phones and WiFi devices in the simulation space because of frequent interruptions of simulator control. For the SOS, it is not necessary to engineer spaces to accommodate *perfect* radio communications. However, understanding that some wireless devices can interfere with each other may help in troubleshooting problems.

In addition to WiFi using 2.4 GHz band, the 5 GHz band (802.11a,ac) does not pass through metal, which can be problematic in many healthcare and simulation settings where metal can be overlaid on walls, and medical equipment and carts can interfere with the signal. Simulation areas that have a divided control room and patient simulator room may have communication hindered if the dividing wall is made of metal. While metal walls are not generally conducive to wireless transmission, the problem may be remedied by changing the devices' operating frequencies to 2.4 GHz. For control rooms that have one-way glass, it should be noted that metal is sometimes a part of the composition of the glass.

Both wireless and wired networks can utilize routers, but *switches* are only used with wired networks, and relatively common in most networks. A router is a device that navigates traffic on a network and typically allows devices to reach beyond the LAN to a larger network such as a company intranet or the Internet. A switch is a device that has anywhere from 3 to 24 ports and accepts Ethernet (RJ-45) cables allowing communication between connected devices (Odum, 2013). Small, consumer wireless routers commonly have a switch built in to allow wired connectivity for devices that do not support WiFi. See Figure 9.1 for basic router/switch configurations.

NETWORK ADDRESSES

In order to allow devices on a network to communicate, the SOS should have an understanding of how to assign a network address. Internet Protocol or IP addresses configured on network devices facilitate data transfer to and from that address. IP addresses can change based on the network architecture and then be reused on other network devices. Private LANs can have hundreds of devices connected and are able to communicate with each other. However, no two devices can have the same IP address without interfering with connectivity with one or both devices. While IP addressing is one of those topics that can quickly go beyond the scope of this chapter, some common addressing schemes and addresses that an SOS may encounter are discussed in subsequent paragraphs.

An IP address serves two purposes: location and identification. The anatomy of an IP address is divided into four octets (e.g. 192.168.1.10). The octets represent a number ranging from 0 to 255. The first three octets are known as a *subnet* (192.168.1.XXX). The last octet typically identifies the *node* (XXX.XXX.XXX.213); a *node* is any device that receives or can be assigned an IP address (Odum, 2013). Therefore, for example, a *node* can be a computer, mobile device, or a server.

This anatomy of an IP address, however, only pertains to IPv4 (IP version 4). This IP addressing protocol does not apply to IPv6 (IP version 6), which is meant to be a replacement for IPv4. However, a` simulation facility will typically use the IPv4 protocol since most simulator manufacturers have not adopted IPv6 protocol (Fig. 9.2).

Basically, a router receives information (a packet) from a node (computer connected to the network) and sends it to another IP address. The destination IP address, like a mail to address on a post envelope, informs routers that exist between the initial node and the destination, where the information (packet) should be sent (Ciampa, 2014). Just as a letter in the postal service would be sent to one distribution center after another, a packet is routed to further networks until it reaches its target destination. Consider the first three octets of the IP address (subnet) as a street address and the last octet (node) as an intended person's name (recipient). The data packet is intended for a particular host on a particular subnet just as a letter could be intended for a particular person in a certain building (Fig. 9.3).

(a)

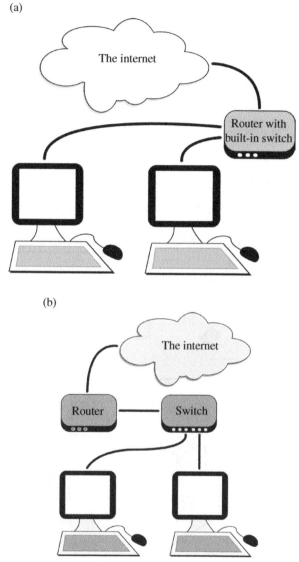

(b)

FIGURE 9.1 Network router with built in switch—(a). Network Switch with separate router—(b).

PUBLIC AND PRIVATE NETWORK ADDRESSING SCHEMES

In order to allow devices, or *nodes*, on a network to pass data packets to other nodes or devices, a basic understanding of addressing schemes is helpful. IP addresses are associated with devices (or nodes). Private (local) IP addresses can change based on the network and are reused for other network nodes. However, *public* IP addresses

An IPv4 address—represented by four numbers separated by periods

Each number represents 8 bits – 8 bits × 4 = 32 bits

194.211.30.101

Network   Node

An IPv6 address—represented by eight groups of hexadecimal digits

Each group represents 2 × 8 bits (16 bits) – 16 bits × 8 = 128 bits

2011:0BD2:7734:A12F:2A01:1002:EB26:0528

FIGURE 9.2   Comparison of the IPv4 and IPv6 address schemas.

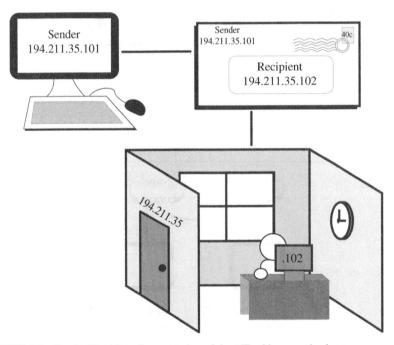

FIGURE 9.3   Sender IP address (computer), recipient IP address, and subnet as represented by three octets. Final octet defines either the sending device or the receiving device.

are usually unique to one device at a time. *Public* IP addresses generally follow a numbering scheme and are purchased or reserved. *Private* LANs can have as many as 4,294,967,296 devices on an IPv4 network. They can be connected to the Internet, but must have a firewall between the LAN and the Internet, to allow only approved traffic to pass between the LAN and the Internet. Each computer may also have a firewall to limit unapproved network traffic, which can further complicate problem

TABLE 9.1 IP Address Numbering Ranges and Schemes

Private IP addresses	These ranges of addresses are reserved and are not routed on the Internet and should only be used on private LANs or LANs connected to the Internet via a router.	10.0.0.0–10.255.255.255 172.16.0.0–172.31.255.255 192.168.0.0–192.168.255.255
Loopback	The *loopback address* is the sender's address for itself. This address is typically used in testing the function of NIC or network connectivity in some way and would not be a valid address to manually configure on a device.	127.0.0.0–127.255.255.255
Reserved	Reserved IP addresses were set aside as IP addressing was developed. The reason these addresses are set aside is not entirely known but there remain a few ranges of address that would not likely be used on a network.	0.0.0.0–0.255.255.255 128.0.0.0–128.0.255.255 191.255.0.0–191.255.255.255 192.0.0.0–192.0.0.255 223.255.255.0–223.255.255.255

identification. Common IP addresses used for private networking exist, but private networks are unlimited in the IP addresses that are available, since they will not have conflicts with other devices outside of the network. Refer to Table 9.1 for IP address numbering and schemes.

Since there are a finite number of public IP addresses, routers are typically used to connect a LAN with servers and routers on the Internet. Most organizations (such as a university or business) will have a particular range of public IP addresses reserved; this can be represented by an entire subnet or a range inside of a subnet. A router configured as a gateway to the Internet, directing traffic intended for devices beyond the LAN, would be assigned a public IP address. Traffic that originates from a host on the LAN and is intended for devices connected to the LAN will not pass through the router, staying internal; the devices connected to the LAN (behind the router) would likely have private IP addresses (Odum, 2013). This allows a number of devices to utilize a single (or few) public IP address(es). In some cases, cable Internet or DSL customers have access to one public IP address. In order for that customer to connect multiple devices, a router is used.

MANUAL AND AUTOMATIC ASSIGNMENT OF IP ADDRESSES

Many routers and some servers are able to assign IP addresses automatically to connected devices. This is known as DHCP or *Dynamic Host Configuration Protocol*. DHCP is a service that runs on a router or server that assigns each IP address to each connected node. A router or server that performs this service is known as a *DHCP server*. The range of IP addresses assigned is configured on the server (router) and devices must be configured to accept IP addresses from a DHCP server in order to receive an IP address. DHCP is common in end user environments and in the simulation environment. It is helpful in environments where a number of computers will need access to the network, but do not require a specific IP address. A DHCP server will also help avoid IP address conflicts where two hosts have the same IP address. An SOS can expect to see a mix of dynamic (DHCP assigned) and static IP addressing.

One can manually configure a *static IP address* for each node, such as a computer, simulator, or other device. Duplicate IP address conflicts can cause errors in communication and should be avoided. Some network devices must have static IP addresses. In the simulation environment, computers that act as control computers for patient simulators commonly use *static* IP manually assigned addresses so that information can be gathered from the computer by other devices during simulation sessions. One example can be found where a video recording solution will also gather event and learner data from the simulator control computer and index the recorded sessions with participant information and bookmarks.

One of the disadvantages of manually configuring fixed IP addresses to multiple nodes is that the DHCP server can assign a fixed address to another node, even though it has been manually assigned to another node. Manually assigning IP addresses is risky. However, with the assistance of the DHCP server administrator, fixed addresses can be reserved using DHCP services. In order to assign a fixed address to a node, the media access control (MAC) address, which is explained in the next section, must be registered with the DHCP server. DHCP assigned "fixed" addresses provide the best of both worlds; the address will not change, so scripting and configuration will not need to be done manually on each node.

ROADBLOCKS TO CONNECTIVITY

Firewalls use IP addresses, MAC (hardware) addresses, and *ports* to limit traffic. Security concerns are the primary reason for these controls, but an added benefit is freeing up network bandwidth. *MAC* addresses are unique identifiers given to any device that communicates over a network; no two devices will share the same MAC address in the entire world. MAC addresses are divided into six octets (or bytes); MAC address octets are generally separated by colons (e.g. 0e:2a:34:ef:28:a3), but may appear as a single string of numbers and letters without separation, or may have a space between each octet. MAC addresses are not named for any one manufacturer, but help identify a device's manufacturer (i.e. Novell or Dell). MAC addresses are commonly referred to as *physical* or *hardware* addresses.

The detailed configuration of firewalls and discussion of port designations is beyond the scope of this text, but an SOS would be at an advantage to understand the basic operation and purpose of a firewall. Many times, a firewall is running, like a service, on a router. A standalone computer can function as a firewall and separate an entire network from the Internet and other networks in an organization. An SOS could encounter a situation where the firewall is blocking a desirable function of an application or operating system. Manufacturers and software developers have identified such problems and can help the SOS provide a solution.

If there is a performance issue that is resolved by disabling the computer's firewall, the SOS may want to find out which port or address is being blocked. Disabling the firewall entirely should only be used as a temporary diagnostic measure. Instead of disabling the firewall entirely or permanently, the SOS could add an exception to the firewall, allowing specific software or services to access the requested ports. An SOS could also encounter difficulty with corporate firewalls. Many times, an organization will implement a firewall on an entire network that might end up blocking desired traffic in addition to security risks. An SOS familiar with basic firewall terminology and operation would be able to communicate with networking technicians to find a solution to the issue. A common solution would be to request an exception to allow traffic from a specific MAC address or port, which will permit correct network operation.

An SOS should become familiar with various types of wireless security and protocols. WEP, WPA and WPA2 are, by far, the most common encryption methods for wireless networking. WPA2 is often preferred and is, for the most part, the most secure. In the simulation environment, the SOS will need to determine what, if any, security is required on the *wireless local area network* or WLAN. Some patient simulator configurations rely on the use of wireless routers to communicate and the patient simulators may or may not be able to communicate via secured wireless connection.

NETWORK MANAGEMENT CONCEPTS

Domain

In many institutions, management of computers and other devices is accomplished with software systems or devices. Microsoft Windows Server™, with various services enabled, places computers and other network devices in virtual containers. An effective and preferred container is a *domain*. A domain is an organization of networked computers and at least one server that manages a list of users and computers. Within a domain, special folders called *organization units* or OUs allow the network administrator to apply different settings to different computers based on their location in the various organization units. If a user has an account on the domain, that user can log into almost any computer that is on the domain (unless prohibited by system policies). A user's capabilities on the computer and network are determined by the user's account settings on the domain, and subsequently the OU where the computer *object* is located, not the user settings on the individual computers. This contrasts with a *workgroup*.

Workgroup

A workgroup is one or more computers that reside on one LAN and have access to shared folders, files, and some resources. It may include one or more servers, but user permissions are defined at each computer, not by a central server, as in the domain model. All networked Windows computers are either a part of a workgroup or a domain. If a computer is set up as a single, non-networked computer, that computer will have a workgroup all to itself.

Domain or Workgroup   To log in to a computer on a workgroup, one must have an account on that computer. The account settings on one computer may not match the account settings for the same user on another computer. One of the advantages of domain control is consistency in user settings. Another notable advantage commonly seen in the simulation environment is the authentication of enterprise software via domain. If the organization purchases enterprise edition software, such as the Windows operating systems, that software can be authenticated, updated, and managed through the domain. An SOS should be familiar with the parameters of domains such as *user accounts, computer accounts,* and basic management of networks. Typically, an SOS has to consider the benefits and drawbacks of domain control and decide what computers, if any, should be added to a domain. There are some computers that will be used to control elements of the simulation environment and will not have access to a corporate network. That type of computer may be best managed with local accounts and not placed on a domain. The institution's IT department or network administrator can help determine the best approach. The expertise of the SOS should not be discounted, however, as an understanding of the simulation equipment and software will be needed, and should help inform the IT team.

The Server/Client Relationship   One technology found in current simulation environments that relies on database management would be an inventory control solution. If the simulation center has an extensive amount of supplies in a number of labs, a need may exist to track these supplies in order to keep records, charge customers, and make reorders. Ideally, this type of technology would hold information on a server and could be modified by several network computers (clients). In order for users to be able to log in and access this system, *a user database* must be established. Responsibility for inventory management may fall to the SOS, as is described in the CHSOS manual as part of Domain III.

Another example of a client–server relationship can be found in a common *web client* interface. Video recording solutions can utilize this type of interface for the management and use of the video capture system. A web browser, acting as a *client,* can initiate a relationship with the video capture *server.* The user can then access the videos on the server or conduct administrative duties via the client interface. The *server* would continue to house the information and files, essentially "serving" the requested information to the *client*; the user can access this information through the web interface. *Client–server* models can take many forms. The operations specialist should understand these basic concepts.

SOS FOUNDATIONS FROM THE WORLD OF AUDIOVISUAL TECHNOLOGY

Audiovisual technology is a field that is becoming less and less distinct from IT. As digital video and audio become standard and AV needs are addressed with IT solutions, the lines between the two fields become more ambiguous. For the purposes of outlining the responsibilities of the SOS, the two fields will be considered separate. Note that the CHSOS blueprint categorizes audiovisual competencies as part of Domain II, along with IT competencies. The efforts of the SOS are frequently employed in capturing simulation for the purpose of review, debriefing, research, and teaching in addition to supporting the presentation and execution of simulation.

Analog and Digital Transmission

Analog   Light and sound, in their most basic forms, are *waves*. The intensity, frequency, and number of waves determine what the eyes or ears perceive. Analog communication is the same concept. Some type of sensor (e.g. a microphone diaphragm) converts sound or light waves to an electromagnetic signal and transmits through some type of medium, typically a wire. Cameras have light sensors and microphones have diaphragms that range in style and purpose but the overall goal is the same: information is interpreted and transmitted in electromagnetic form. This process allows an analog signal to be carried to a particular destination. For example, a person controlling a manikin from a control room can speak to a student who is interacting with the simulated patient. A microphone is used to capture that sound (waves) and transmit to an amplifier that uses the electromagnetic interpretation of the sound to send a powerful signal to a speaker that then projects that signal as a louder version of the original sound.

Digital   Digital transmission is yet another interpretation of the electromagnetic waves. A device, such as a computer sound card, accepts the input of an electromagnetic, analog signal and then creates, or codes, a description of the sound. A device that can convert analog signal to digital information is called an ADC or *analog to digital converter* (Hass, 2003). These devices are generally designed to interpret digital information and produce an analog version as well; this function is known as a *digital to analog converter* (DAC). Consider the example of the person controlling the manikin and speaking as the patient. Suppose the interaction between the student and the simulated patient is being recorded by a computer. This process occurs when the microphone captures the sound and sends the electromagnetic signal to a device such as an audio interface card. The interface card, or ADC, codes the signal as a digital file. The file is a digital interpretation of the analog signal heard by the interface card and can be saved to the computer's hard drive. When it is time to play the file back and listen to the recording, the computer will send the digital file to the audio interface card. The card, performing the DAC process, will interpret the digital information from the file, and transmit an analog signal, or sound, as an output (Hass, 2003).

CODEC   There are standards by which analog information is coded. These standards result in the different file types for audio, video, and pictures. A CODEC is responsible for gathering information on a source and then arranging that information so that the file can be read by a device with that same CODEC. CODEC is a contraction for *code-decode*; functionally, a CODEC is program that accepts a digital media file and compresses the file in a different format or file type. There are hundreds of file types for pictures, audio, and video; in order to decode or read a file, the device must have the CODEC related to that file type. Some file types are not cross-compatible and some are specific to certain programs. A list of common multimedia file types is listed in the table below. Keep in mind that a particular software vendor may elect to use a custom or *proprietary* CODEC. If a video does not playback with its normally associated application, a plug-in may be needed to add the correct CODEC for that application.

Refer to Appendix 4 for common formats of files, including multimedia such as video, images, and audio.

Videography and Photography

Video and photos are often used for the purposes of documentation, promotion, and instruction and are commonplace in the simulation environment. The SOS would be at an advantage knowing the basic operation of cameras. Advanced use of digital single-lens reflex (DSLR) cameras is not necessary, especially when the devices have automatic mode. Cameras typically allow the user to change shutter speed, shutter opening, gain, and a myriad of other settings. Automatic mode allows the camera to determine the best setting automatically and generally produces acceptable results. If the simulation environment relies on video recordings, the site may have (or need) permanent cameras integrated with a recording solution. PTZ (pan-tilt-zoom) cameras are typically mounted and have the ability to pan, tilt, and zoom remotely. This function is convenient in places where monitoring and recording is frequent and setting up cameras on tripods would be time consuming and take up usable floor space. Permanent cameras can be wired to send video signal to a CODEC or to a video switcher and routed to other devices such as monitor displays.

Common Connections/Hardware for Audiovisual Solutions   Analog audio connectors are common and necessary in the simulation environment. See the table below for common audio connections and example of uses in the simulation environment.

Refer to Appendix 3 for examples of audio connections and how they might be used in the simulation environment. Video connections are not only necessary for computer operations but for camera and multimedia solutions found in many simulation environments. Refer to Appendix 3 for examples of video connections and how they might be used in the simulation environment.

Signal Chain Troubleshooting   Video and audio transmissions exist in "chains." There are almost always one or more destinations for every source. Consider that a computer video card is a *source*. A common configuration: The signal must travel from the computer's video card, through a cable (possibly a VGA or DVI), and finally to a monitor or *display*. Figure 9.4 illustrates a more complex configuration for a camera recording solution.

Note that this example is merely one type of configuration that can be found in simulation environments. This example seeks to present the analogy of a "chain" so that an operations specialist may begin troubleshooting at one end or the other. Many current configurations will not include a video switcher. Following this model to troubleshoot an issue may still be helpful even though the configuration does not resemble this example.

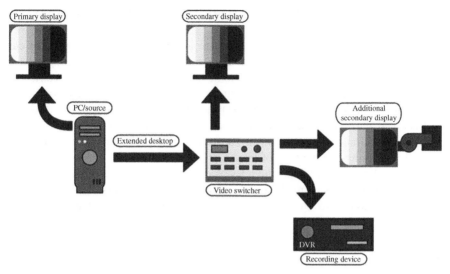

FIGURE 9.4   Example of an A/V configuration with complex signal chain routing.

Troubleshooting with this type of environment can be simplified by starting at one end of the signal chain. If the video is not successfully being recorded, an SOS could start with an inspection of the source and proceed through the chain until the problem "link" is identified. Working from the source, the SOS should make sure the power is connected and turned on. Verify that the camera is connected to the switcher with a video cable, and the signal is getting to the switcher is covering the first portion of the signal chain. Once the SOS is convinced the signal is not hindered up to that point, the next step is to move on to the next section of the chain. This process could require disconnecting and reconnecting devices and cables in order to test operation with another device (i.e. connect a different camera to the connection belonging to the camera in question). This process is helpful when it is unclear where to begin troubleshooting. At other times, a troublesome device has continual problems and is the known "weak link" of a system and can serve as starting point of the trouble-shooting process.

RESOLUTION, BANDWIDTH, AND FREQUENCY RELATED TO A/V COMMUNICATION/TRANSMISSION

An SOS would not be expected to configure advanced settings on devices in an audiovisual configuration but may find the terminology and concepts useful. Video devices will accept a range of *refresh rates*. Refresh rate is the rate at which a digital video signal is repeated to a device. Some displays, video interface cards, and other video devices will not be able to "see" a video signal if its refresh rate is beyond what is compatible. This is an important aspect to consider when configuring AV systems utilizing digital video components.

SOS FOUNDATIONS FROM THE WORLD OF THEATER AND DRAMA

From the worlds of theater and drama, there are a number of concepts that can be applied to simulation in healthcare education that may have gone unrecognized or overlooked. The SOS may be expected to be involved in incorporating theatrical or façade elements into the instructional context. Many times these elements are generated in impromptu situations and the SOS must develop skills without structured instructional curricula. These elements are generally exacted in order to create realism in the simulated environment. The need for this realism depends on the type of clinical training and the type of learner or participant involved. An example of a type of simulation that demands high levels of realism is *disaster response training*. Emergency medical personnel can be trained to respond to disasters using mock disaster situations and subsequent patient simulation sessions that incorporate realistic injuries and wounds.

Vocal Façades

Clinical education, in particular, relies on the use of patient simulators to teach students how to interact with real patients. This can be successful in an environment where the patient talks and responds like a human being. The simulator operator remains out of sight, but through an AV system or proximity to the simulator, can hear what the "patient" hears and can talk through the simulator.

An interesting technique that adds to the façade element is the use of a voice modulator to make the operator's voice sound like the gender of the "patient." A voice modulator or *vocoder* is a device or software that alters the sound passing through a microphone, in this case, to sound like the opposite sex. This technique is not always needed, but can be an impressive and effective one.

Pitch and Formant   Two qualities of a person's speech affect vocalization; these are pitch and *formant*. The pitch difference between men and women's voices are apparent, but *formant* is less noticeable, but important. The length of male vocal tract is longer than a female's, resulting in a slower *formant*. *Formant* is also known as the acoustic resonance of a voice and helps describe the formation of sounds by the human vocal tract; this formation of speech gives a voice character and depth. The SOS should know that an effective vocal modulator, or *vocoder*, will not be able to perfectly modify this vocal property, but can come very close. Typically, a sound effect like this is implemented toward the source side of the signal chain, right after the microphone.

Moulage, Make-up, and the "Health" of Simulation Technology

Chapter 5 explains the concept of moulage more thoroughly, but an SOS should be concerned about the health of the technology that exists in the simulation environment. Many patient simulators have simulated skin that will stain or scar easily. As an SOS, it is easy to forget that some simulated parts of a body are not as resilient as the real thing and cannot heal or be washed like the human body. Moulage describes the process of applying simulated wounds and injuries to manikins (or actors). This process is very helpful in creating a realistic simulation space, but presents a risk to technology when dyes, fluids, and glues are used. The SOS must carefully review the user manual and research the ingredients in moulage supplies to consider what might be harmful to a simulator to ensure that manufacturer warranties are not voided.

SOS FOUNDATIONS FROM THE WORLD OF ACADEMIA

The fields of education and academia offer an array of ideas that are evident in the world of an SOS. The following concepts are relevant to the work of the SOS at a basic level:

- Identification of differences between established instructional strategies, contexts, and goals.
- Identification of learner abilities and needs.
- Identification and definition of performance objectives and how they relate to instructional goals.
- Processes for developing, modifying, and implementing curriculum.

Instructors or managers can expect the SOS to make decisions about scenario components and learning methods based on prior experience. The SOS may be expected to advise educators and managers on the appropriate simulation modality to achieve certain goals. The SOS who has appropriate experience or academic preparation can be an asset with lesson planning and instructional design when requested to do so. Typically, the SOS must rely on the subject matter expert for guidance.

Healthcare curricula in higher education environments (and elsewhere) exist in a context that considers class schedules, instructor availability, prerequisites, learner course load, and a myriad of other factors. Scheduling of simulation-based education may be forced to work around these factors and cannot be changed immediately without appropriate collaboration. An SOS should be aware of these factors when scheduling simulations sessions.

SOS FOUNDATIONS FROM THE WORLD OF HEALTHCARE

Concepts from the field of healthcare directly influence the types of technology used in the simulation environment. The focus of the specific healthcare simulation program will determine terminology and concepts that must be learned by the SOS. Chapter 6 goes into greater depth on this topic, but some of these are:

- Cardiac arrhythmias (irregular heart rhythms): Intermediate and advanced patient simulators simulate these rhythms so that they can be heard, felt at pulse areas, and reflected on patient monitors.

- Pharmacology (medications and their interactions): A patient simulator may indicate a physiological response to a certain type of medicine, administration route, or dosage.
- Medicine administration (route and conditions that determine how a patient receives medicine): Patient simulators are designed to accommodate most medicine administration routes and some even have mechanisms to detect when and how a particular type of medication is administered.
- Anatomy and physiology (the structure and function of the parts of the human body): Patient simulators are designed to be as anatomically correct as possible, from bone structure to arteries and veins.
- Health assessment (the initial examination of a patient by a healthcare professional): This is a process that is generally similar across healthcare professions and is one of the primary skills students are expected to learn.
- In-hospital and pre-hospital environments: Pre-hospital is any environment in which a patient would exist before they reach a hospital; a corn field and an ambulance are both pre-hospital environments. In-hospital refers to environments in which healthcare professionals perform duties inside a hospital.
- Hospital personnel and departments (hierarchy, roles, and departments in the hospital): Many hospital roles and departments (e.g. MD, ED, and PT) are referenced in healthcare education, even in a specific field such as nursing or respiratory therapy.

CONCLUSION: CONTEXT MATTERS

There are numerous types of knowledge, skills, and attributes (KSAs) from which the SOS could benefit. But such KSAs vary, to some extent, depending on a number of factors. After considering the lengthy list of skills that could potentially comprise the SOS job description, one should remember that the actual expectations of the SOS will not likely look like the summation of this chapter or even the full CHSOS blueprint. Some KSAs and expectations discussed in this chapter might be omitted from SOS responsibilities and expectations at a particular simulation program. Equally true, some items NOT described in this chapter may be added to the expectations of a program's SOS. Overall, two primary factors will influence the scope of the SOS role.

Mission and the SOS

First, the center's mission will shape the responsibilities of the SOS as well as other roles in the program. Consequently, the specific healthcare focus of a program will shape an SOS's responsibilities. An SOS working in the respiratory therapy department of a community college will need a different set of healthcare-related skills when compared with an SOS in a baccalaureate-nursing program. Nasogastric tube insertion, for example, is a skill that would be simulated to help train nurses, but would be unlikely in a center dedicated to respiratory therapy.

The second characteristic that will shape the responsibilities of an SOS is the type of institution where the simulation program resides. For example, an SOS could have the support of an IT team that will determine and support the use of routers and switches. This type of resource, leaving the SOS to focus on the educational- and healthcare-related responsibilities aforementioned, could satisfy the specific responsibilities discussed earlier as it relates to networking, database management. Conversely, an SOS could work closely with instructors who are responsible for the designing the learning opportunities, create scenarios, and teaching learners. In this situation, the SOS would likely satisfy most technical responsibilities and possess only enough healthcare-related skills to communicate and understand needs in the simulated environment. Either one of these examples will still need foundational knowledge, skills, and attributes in areas exist in others, but will have their responsibilities essentially shaped by the presence or absence of other employees in the organization.

The role of the SOS is not specific to any one position, but refers to anyone that specializes in simulation operations associated with healthcare education. Many of those who are in such a role began with experience in at least one of the five foundational fields with limited or no experience in the other fields. While it is important to understand the scope of the knowledge needed, it is not necessary to have achieved mastery in all of the associated fields in the beginning.

This Venn diagram illustrates the concept that the role of SOS is not one formed from a specific area of knowledge but from many knowledge areas (Fig. 9.5).

The role of the SOS is not specific to any one position, but refers to anyone that specializes in the operations of simulation in healthcare education. Many of those who are in the role began with experience in one or more of the five fields with limited or no experience the other fields. While it is important to understand the

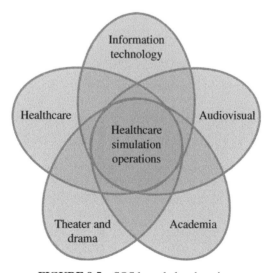

FIGURE 9.5   SOS knowledge domains.

scope of the knowledge needed, it is not necessary to have achieved mastery in all of the associated fields in the beginning. What is also important is a willingness to strive to know as much as possible about all aspects of the role.

REFERENCES

Andrews, J. (2013). *A+ guide to managing and maintaining your PC* (8th ed.). Boston, MA: Cengage Learning.

Ciampa, M. (2014). *CompTIA security+ guide to network security fundamentals* (5th ed.). Boston, MA: Cengage Learning.

Hass, J. (Ed.). (2003). Digital audio. In: *Introduction to computer music* (Vol. *1*). Bloomington, IN: Jacobs School of Music, Indiana University. Retrieved from: http://www.indiana.edu/~emusic/etext/toc.shtml

Odum, W. (2013). *CCNA routing and switching 200-120: Official cert guide library* (1st ed.). Indianapolis, IN: Pearson Education.

10

PROGRAMMING PATIENT OUTCOMES IN SIMULATION: CONCEPTS IN SCENARIO STANDARDIZATION AND AUTOMATION

H. Michael Young[1] and Valeriy Kozmenko[2]

[1] *Level 3 Healthcare, Mesa, AZ, USA*
[2] *Parry Center for Clinical Skills and Simulation, Sioux Falls, SD, USA*

INTRODUCTION

What *is* a *scenario*? For the purposes of this chapter:

> a *scenario* is a combination of a physiological and/or pathophysiological model of the medical condition and a complex decision-making tree that reflects the patient's response(s) to the various interventions that lead to any number of possible clinical outcomes. Multiple clinical outcomes are the key difference between simulation scenarios, case studies, and standardized patient/participant (SP) cases/scripts.

A *scenario* with multiple possible outcomes that depends on the participant's action has a higher engagement potential than a static case study and many SP encounters. Scenarios allow for experiences that enable the participants to determine the appropriateness of their action, or inaction, via the feedback demonstrated by patient outcomes. The approach in which a participant experiments, takes alternative actions,

Healthcare Simulation: A Guide for Operations Specialists, First Edition.
Edited by Laura T. Gantt and H. Michael Young.
© 2016 John Wiley & Sons, Inc. Published 2016 by John Wiley & Sons, Inc.

and observes the result *is the major advantage of a scenario over a static case study*. Therefore, a scenario is an *outcome-based, event-driven teaching* (OET) *concept*. There are up to two roles that are engaged in the operation of a scenario: *facilitator* and *operator*. At times this may be one person performing both roles simultaneously. The difference is the facilitator is typically the subject matter expert (SME). Primarily, each role is determined whether the person is operating the simulator or making the decisions based on an assessment of the participant's performance. If both the facilitator and operator roles are performed by two individuals, most likely, the facilitator "gets the credit" (Gantt, 2012, p. 585).

OUTCOME-BASED, EVENT-DRIVEN TEACHING (OET): OUTCOME VERSUS THE EVENT

There are two key words in the OET concept: the *outcome* and the *event*. The *outcome* is comprised of the feedback mechanism that informs the learner on whether the action was correct/successful or incorrect/detrimental. The *event* is the driving force that keeps the scenario moving forward and provides learning opportunities. The *events* or *actions* that a participant may or may not take pose both the *advantage* and the *challenge* of OET.

The Event and Outcome Relationship

The "event" is the *decision point* for the participant, where an *action* results in a specific *outcome*. The *live improvised operation* (LIO) (aka "on the fly") and the standardized automation operation (SAO) methods rely on these two concepts, but the SAO method has a predetermined outcome incorporated during the design process, while the LIO method depends on the facilitator's discernment as the scenario unfolds. With the SAO method, the scenario designer identifies those *events* that must or must not take place during the scenario, then defines the appropriate outcomes. Each "event" introduces an opportunity for the participant, or is precipitated by the participant.

There are two kinds of events in SAO: *passive* and *reflexive*. A *passive* event is defined as those events that are precipitated by the internal processes of the simulator (patient) where an outcome will occur whether the participant addresses the cause or not. A reflexive event is characterized by the actions of an external intervention or action. The participant performs an intervention (action) which results in a predetermined *outcome*. In the following example, we can identify several possibilities on whether an event is *passive* or *reflexive*.

If a "patient" presents with pulseless ventricular tachycardia (pulseless VT) at some point in the scenario, regardless of learner action, this outcome is simultaneously an event and an outcome. It is an *event* because the programming has initiated the pulseless VT at a predetermined point in the scenario. So, the *event* is *passive*. An appropriate intervention by the scenario participant is to administer an unsynchronized shock of

200 joules using a biphasic defibrillator. However, this is also an *event* that is precipitated by the participant, not the programming. However, whether or not the administration of a shock can be construed as *reflexive* or *passive* depends on how the simulator is programmed. If the shock itself automatically precipitates cardiac conversion to normal sinus rhythm, then the simulator programming has determined the outcome (sinus rhythm), and is still *passive* from the perspective of the operator.

Regardless of the simulator platform, *events* and *outcomes* are important components in scenario design, and consequently are important in scenario programming.

Whether through LIO or SAO methods, the OET approach allows the scenario designer to define more than one path that a scenario might take based on the interventions (events/actions) performed by the participants. Thus, an effective simulation scenario should allow for multiple possible outcomes that depend on the physiological and pathophysiological changes of a given medical condition and the actions of the participant(s).

The OET concept-based scenario design provides a strong foundation whether implemented through SAO or LIO. The SAO method can be associated with the phrase *programmed* (or *preprogrammed*) *scenario*. However, not all programmed scenarios are standardized, nor do all have an appropriate level of automation. The LIO method does not necessarily mean that the scenario is standardized or not standardized. Implementation of both the SAO and LIO methods are *outcome-based* and *event-driven* teaching/training (OET) methods of scenario design.

Develop for Experts, Adjust for Novices   Scenario design can occur in a way that it is educationally sound and useful for novices, intermediate, and expert levels of participants. This can be achieved by designing the scenario that would be challenging, realistic, and appropriate for even the most seasoned participants. For the less experienced participant, the complexity of the scenario can be designed with additional prompts and subtle hints during scenario facilitation. This well-tested approach allows reuse of a scenario for various levels of participants without the need to design a different scenario for each level—programmed or not. In addition, the "develop for experts, adjust for novices" approach forces the scenario designer to think about how the scenario will be implemented and debriefed.

OET: Live Improvised Operation (On the Fly)

In the LIO method of scenario facilitation, the facilitator observes the *actions* of the participant(s), decides what should be the *outcome* for each *action*, and as operator adjusts the simulator's physiologic response in *real time*. Consequently, the authors have chosen to use the term LIO to describe this approach. A more popular term for LIO is "on the fly." "On the fly" does not clearly describe the expectations and methodology implemented in the LIO method, so the authors have introduced new terminology that clarifies the concept and improves communication between professionals.

One of the main benefits of the LIO method is its flexibility. However, it comes at the cost of requiring an SME to be present during the scenario session in order to determine the appropriate outcome for each participant's intervention (or lack thereof) (Slone & Lampotang, 2015, p. 185). In general, clinical faculty have busy schedules. Between their clinical and teaching responsibilities, adding simulation to the curriculum may then require the SME's presence in the simulation lab. Often, limited funding for many undergraduate clinical programs precludes their educators and staff from attending simulation conferences and training events where best practices in healthcare simulation are established and taught. This often negatively affects the quality of simulation-based teaching.

Additionally, the LIO method is inherently inconsistent and has potential for bias. The temptation to alter scenario conditions based on a variety of reasons and rationale is very high. Sometimes, the facilitator sees a "new" opportunity to enhance the learner's experience, but when this occurs, the potential for changing the focus away from the original objectives is likely. Consequently, learners and even the facilitator can negatively affect the scenario if participants think that their altered experience resulted in poor performance. In an effort to ensure that the scenario remains focused on achieving its original learning objectives, standardization of the scenario must become a priority.

LIO and Physiologic Model-based Simulators   Some simulators, such as CAE's *human patient simulator*, have built-in physiologic models that allow for improved simulation of various physiologic and pathophysiologic processes. Using the simulator's control software, the facilitator/operator needs to change physiologic parameters of the patient simulator that, in turn, changes its vital signs. For example, to change a "patient's" blood pressure, one needs to alter myocardial contractility and systemic vascular resistance; two major determining factors for blood pressure. Often, a physiologic model is more of an obstacle than a benefit when the operation of the simulator is done via the LIO method alone. For example, when myocardial contractility and systemic vascular resistance are changed, it is impossible to predict what would be the resulting blood pressure (Slone & Lampotang, 2015). The scenario designer needs to experiment with these two parameters and program them into the scenario beforehand. Consequently, the LIO mode, in this example, will not be practical.

OET: Standardized Automated Operation (SAO)

The second method of simulator operation utilizes the built-in programming tools provided by the simulator manufacturer to automate (with or without manual override) scenarios that have the capacity to:

- simulate physiologic changes of a given condition,
- recognize participant actions,
- correctly interpret them, and
- generate a physiologic response.

This method allows the operator to translate every decision-making step (event) into the software's code to enable the outcomes of a simulator to be operator-independent. In this case, the scenario outcomes are the result of their interaction of the participants with the "patient" rather than an instructor superimposing his or her own judgment on the outcomes of the scenario. Slone and Lampotang (2015, p. 186) refer to this approach as "state-based modeling." However, this may be an oversimplification depending on the complexity of the actual programming strategies used. Many approach programming from a *state-based* perspective, but the authors here are proposing that the connection between scenario design and scenario programming go beyond individual states, or even the transition between them. The most complex part of this approach is for the scenario designer to:

- anticipate *all* possible actions that might be taken (or not taken) by each participant and
- program the simulator to respond appropriately to each action.

To achieve this, the scenario designer must not only have access to the *treatment protocols* for a given medical condition, but also know the capabilities, possible knowledge gaps, and misconceptions of the participants. To ensure that all alternative routes through the scenario are anticipated and correctly programmed, the scenario designer/operator needs to have several test runs of the scenario, making changes as new insights about the scenario are discovered.

SIMULATION OPERATIONS SPECIALIST, SUBJECT-MATTER EXPERT, AND PROGRAMMING

In order to incorporate programmed responses, the scenario designer and the scenario programmer need *not* be the same person. For example, an SME can collaborate with a technician, or *simulation operations specialist* (SOS). In essence, "two heads are better than one." The educator (SME) ensures that the design of the scenario is accurate and meets defined objectives for the appropriate participants. The operations specialist can translate the scenario design into scenario programming. Inevitably, the process of programming may raise new questions that the designer did not take into account. The most common oversight in a scenario design is exclusion of key information: "what if the participants do not take an expected action?" The SOS should alert the scenario designer on any oversights and await the response. Both designer and programmer may offer solutions. The scenario designer needs to accept that the SOS may become the "SME" in respect to programming, and rely on the programmer to find the most appropriate method to program the scenario—as long as it conforms to the scenario design. Ultimately, the scenario designer is responsible for the accuracy of the scenario design and the results of the programming, but the SOS is an important part of the process, and frees the educator from the tedious task of programming in favor of other duties that only an educator can do. Scenario design has a direct correlation to scenario programming. Whether the scenario designer also programs the scenario or utilizes others on the operations team, understanding the major concepts in both scenario design and programming is critical to a successful outcome.

SAO: SCENARIO DESIGN/PROGRAMMING CONCEPTS

Professional Cultures and Scenario Design Collaboration

Different specialties reside in different cultures and impose specific ways of thinking within these communities of practice. For example, a computer programmer is very accustomed to think in terms of "If this, then that; repeat." Often a clinician and an SOS perceive the same situation very differently.

For example, a team consisting of a clinical educator and SOS is developing a malignant hyperthermia scenario. Setting the stage for the malignant hyperthermia scenario …

- … the clinician says to the SOS, "This is an 8-year old boy. The participants will induce him into anesthesia with sevoflurane."
- The SOS asks, "What if they use a different method of induction into anesthesia?"
- The clinician replies, "No, this is what they usually do."

As clinicians become more experienced in simulation design, they eventually come to understand that *the participants will be making the decisions* during the scenario, NOT *the clinical faculty*. The clinician inevitably comes to realize that *all possible* actions that the *participants* might take MUST be anticipated rather than just the most expected actions. As the clinician and the SOS grow in their knowledge of each other's specialty and understand the mechanisms of how all parties think and make decisions, the gap closes.

Three types of people are typically involved in developing and programming scenarios: (i) clinical SMEs, who know how patients receive treatment in real life; (ii) educators, who know how to teach people; and (iii) technologists, who know how to work with simulator software. An SME and educator are often the same individual, which reduces some of the challenge. Still, those three tribes have their own specialized knowledge, concepts, and language that are associated with a *way of thinking* that is hard to understand for people outside each camp. If these individuals stay in their own silos and fail to learn from the others, problems (or bad scenarios) are inevitable. For example:

A clinician with limited experience in simulation is enthusiastic about writing a scenario. He describes the scenario to the simulation operations specialist, "The patient is in the ER because of unstable atrial fibrillation and chest pain. The participants will cardiovert him and take him to the cath lab where a major vessel is perforated during stenting and the patient develops hemorrhagic shock."

For this scenario to take the anticipated path, the participants need to (i) recognize the rhythm, (ii) correctly treat the patient with synchronized cardioversion, and (iii) decide to take the patient to cardiac catheterization lab. The problem is that developing an internal bleed due to vessel perforation is dependent on the participants' own actions (taking patient to cath lab) and may or may not happen. The clinician has not clarified if there will be another team awaiting in the cath lab, or if the perforation is only assumed, with no action being necessary from the primary group. Unless this scenario is a scene from *ER*, it is not likely the same team that has stabilized the patient for the cath lab.

CONFUSION IN SIMULATION DESIGN
PROGRAMMING TERMINOLOGY

The difficulty of programming a scenario is complicated further by a lack of terminology standardization among individuals in the simulation community. The following concepts have different implications for programming scenarios, so it is important for both the scenario designer and programmer to have a common language.

Scenario

Ironically, one of the most confusing terms in the general simulation community is "scenario." Aside from the definition of *scenario* provided at the beginning of this chapter, a *scenario* is a computer file (programming) that is loaded to control the outcomes of a simulation session. For others, it is the clinical content of the simulation session (scenario design). For others, the words "scenario" and "simulation" are interchangeable. Another term has been introduced in recent years that is also attributed to the concept of a *scenario* but in the context of pedagogy: *simulation-based experiences* (SBE). In this case a "standardized simulation design provides a framework for developing effective SBE" (Lioce et al., 2015, para. 8). Regardless of the contextual meaning, both Laerdal and Gaumard see *scenario* as a **single thread** of potential outcomes, regardless if they are referring to programming code or scenario design. In contrast, the CAE simulator is capable of running several simulation *scenarios* (programming) simultaneously—otherwise known to programmers as **multithreading**. For example, consider that the primary scenario program emulates *hypertensive crisis*. A second *scenario* (programming) emulates anaphylactic shock because of the patient's contact with latex; this part of the programming is dormant until the exposure to latex occurs. Both *scenarios* interact with each other based on the physiologic engine built into the simulator's design. *Technically*, two programmed scenarios are running at the same time, but their interaction is one scenario for the prescribed session. If the operator is launching several programmed scenarios based on predefined triggers, in reality, the combination of more than one scenario (program) is still just one scenario (design) on a CAE simulator.

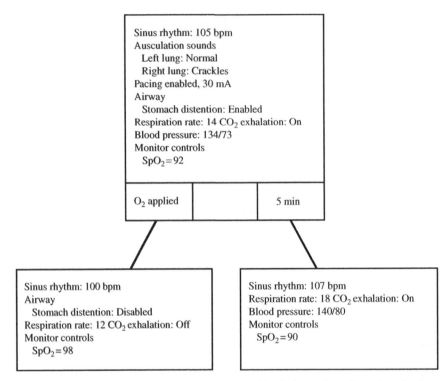

FIGURE 10.1   State/frame/node represents the physiological snapshot of a patient simulator; while they appear differently, the concepts are similar.

Scenario Snapshots: States, Frames, and Nodes   A *state* represents a snapshot of the patient's presented physiological vital parameters, whether presented on a vitals monitor or palpation, observation, or auscultation. For example, CAE calls these physiologic snapshots "states." Each *state* represents various physiological snapshots. On the other hand, Laerdal represents each snapshot using a "frame" in the programming interface (Slone & Lampotang, 2015). Gaumard presents these snapshots as a *node* in its scenario interface. Conceptually, there is very little difference between a *state, frame*, and a *node* (Fig. 10.1).

Trend   A *trend* is understood as a particular or general direction (tendency), like a trend of events. There are two types of trends: (i) historical and (ii) future. A *historical* trend is a matter of record, and unchangeable. However, a *future trend* is interpolated based on the historical trend and is presumptive at best. In the world of simulation scenario programming, a *future trend* can be just as sure as a historical trend. For example, a patient monitor records the trends of the patient's heart rate, pulse oximetry, blood pressure, and temperature, among a variety of other parameters. A clinician can evaluate the *historical trend* of the patient and make assumptions if the patient's outcome is improving or getting worse. In a programmed scenario, a "trend" refers to future trends of physiological outcomes defined over time, and allows for peaks and valleys in the scenario. The simulator operator can see *future trends* convert to *historical trends* right before their eyes as the scenario progresses.

Trends are components within a scenario programming interface that enable the programmer to define what the patient vital signs will be during the scenario. A simple trend defines one or more vital parameters as starting at one metric, changing over time to the determined outcome. In other words, a trend can be programmed to start at an initial SpO_2 level—say 92—and rise *over time* by an additional five points. If *time* is 5 minutes, and the resulting outcome is 97, the programming will automatically do the work for the operator. The trend capability resides in the simulator's scenario programming software. This is an example of a *relative trend* that adjusts a parameter from whatever point in the scenario and takes it up by points, not to a specific number. In contrast, a *fixed trend* is where a parameter that is at one value jumps to the next without any transition time. Of the two types of trends, the relative trend is more realistic.

Trending can occur independently of the programmed scenario (SAO) using the features built into the simulator control interface. However, this takes the operator's attention away from observing the scenario participants, especially as more parameters are being trended. Therefore, in order to maintain operator/facilitator focus on the learners, it is better to have a trend *programmed* to do the changes *automatically*. Each trend can represent a single parameter (such as heart rate) or multiple parameters (heart rate, SpO_2, respiratory rate, and blood pressure, etc.). A *trend* is a critical component of the automation of patient vitals because it reduces operator distractions and improves standardization of the scenario.

As stated, either a trend is programmed to assume a specific value (or metrics) at its start and end, or the *trend* can start the parameter value from whatever state the simulator is at when the trend is launched. In a programmed scenario (SAO), for example, the patient simulator's induction into anesthesia paralyzes the patient who is then placed on mechanical ventilation by the participants. The initial end-tidal CO_2 might be at 35–38 mmHg and then it will change over time (relative trend) to a certain number based on the minute ventilation rate. The programming of this trend starts the trend at a baseline that represents whatever is defined in the state/frame/node as the patient's initial vital signs. Alternatively, for example, a trend can be programmed to change the blood pressure and the heart rate after epinephrine administration. No matter what the initial blood pressure and heart rate, these parameters will increase by the specific predetermined numbers depending on the given dose of epinephrine (Fig. 10.2).

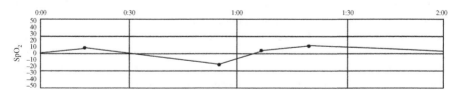

FIGURE 10.2　A trend can include more than one parameter. In this example only the SpO_2 parameter is illustrated. In combination with additional parameter trends, multiple parameters can be automated in concert.

Trigger A *trigger* is a predefined event that launches one or more automated processes in a scenario. A trend can be launched at the outset of a scenario and programmed to run the length of the entire scenario, even if no interventions are administered during the scenario. In this situation, the trigger is the initiation of the scenario itself. The trend runs for the predetermined duration, and will automatically change the vitals as programmed. The *trigger* can also be an event that is programmed to launch a trend. For example, a trend can be programmed to start when the O_2 mask is placed on the patient, so the administration of oxygen is the trigger for the trend to raise the SpO_2 level by five points over 5 minutes.

In Gaumard's scenario programming interface, triggers are *paths*. Each *path* is a predefined trigger that links one node to another node (state, frame). Laerdal's scenario programming interface calls the *trigger* an *event*. CAE HPS software does not use a specific word for trigger. On the CAE interface, the scenario designer programs a transition to define the *condition* to be met (the trigger) and the outcome. The trigger as a *concept* is consistent regardless of the manufacturer's preferred terminology.

Handler A scenario programming component unique to Laerdal's programming interface is the *handler*. A handler is probably the most flexible method for controlling how triggers translate to new outcomes. As a scenario programmer's skills evolve, the handler becomes the preferred method of making triggers/events available anywhere during an advanced scenario; this allows the operator to initiate the trigger, or allows the simulator's features to trigger a trend or other outcome automatically at any time during the scenario.

Threshold One of the risks of automating parameter outcomes with trends is that the programming elevates or drops patient vital signs beyond what would normally be expected or desired. This happens when a learner waits too long to administer an appropriate medication and an additional participant error is introduced that forces the parameters to become exaggerated. Most advanced simulator models enable the programmer to set thresholds so that vitals are constrained to remain within a specific range.

For example, after several sessions of operating an SAO-based chronic obstructive pulmonary disease (COPD) scenario, the programmer received several complaints from facilitators/operators that the patient often "dies" during the scenario, requiring them to manually override respiratory arrest. When asked what the conditions were at the time of the "death" the operators recounted that the scenario participants continued to increase oxygen volume. The scenario's programming was designed to launch a trend to lower respiratory rate each time oxygen was increased. However, in extreme conditions, students failed to identify that their actions were the cause of the cessation of respiration. To prevent complete respiratory arrest of the scenario's patient, a *threshold* was set so that the respiratory rate did not get any lower than four breaths per minute. This satisfied the facilitators/operators, as it was no longer necessary to override the trend that was lowering the respiratory rate.

PROMPTS A good simulation scenario should have built-in mechanisms, or *prompts*, to guide participants in the right direction should they need subtle hints or lose their way. For example, if participants (learners) do not recognize that a "patient" with atrial fibrillation is unstable (blood pressure 80/40 mmHg), and if participants consider controlling the heart rate with a beta blocker, the "patient" can tell participants "my normal blood pressure is 160/100 mmHg." Hopefully, this will guide the participants in the right direction (Dieckmann, Lippert, Glavin, & Rall, 2010).

Prompts can come in various forms. Certainly, the "patient" can communicate with his caregiver about what he is experiencing as a way to give the learner insight into making the appropriate decision and acting on it. However, other prompting methods might include the use of a confederate (or *standardized participant*). If the learner does not notice, for example, that the patient's blood pressure is dropping, and the patient is asleep or unconscious, a "family member" can ask the healthcare provider (participant/learner) "is 80/45 alright?" while pointing to the patient vital signs monitor. Whether the *prompt* comes from the patient, a confederate, or staged clues in the room (such as candy wrappers in the room of a diabetic patient who is complaining of feeling bad), the prompt is an important component to utilize in the design and in some cases, the programming, of the scenario.

Usually, programming a simulation scenario is done with a particular method of facilitation in mind (Lioce et al., 2015, para. 155). Consider a hypothetical scenario of a burned victim with smoke inhalation and a compromised airway. A high priority intervention would be to protect the airway by endotracheal intubation. What if the participants (learners) …

- do not recognize the patient's compromised airway?
- are not able to perform intubation?
- attempt to intubate without sedating the patient?

In developing this scenario, the designer needs to decide whether the "patient" is permitted to "die" as the result of a participant's lethal mistake. How will the operator address other mistakes during the scenario? For example, if participants attempt to intubate a conscious patient, a confederate can *prompt* the participants by describing the patient as agitated and is fighting intubation efforts (since a simulator is unable to demonstrate this behavior). Thus, the structure of the scenario is determined by the ground rules of how simulation activities will be performed. Since different institutions and educators have different teaching approaches, the same scenario could be a perfect tool for one educator and completely inappropriate for another. In like manner, a scenario may be an appropriate experience for one group of participants, and inappropriate for another group. This makes developing one's own scenario a better approach than using commercially available or peer distributed scenarios.

For example, in 2004, Drs. Wilks and Kozmenko were invited to present by the Society of Hospitalists to showcase a particular patient simulator. The presenters had designed and programmed a scenario of a post-op patient complaining of pain, with the assumption that the nurse (as portrayed by the participant) gives the "patient" an excessive amount of morphine. Consequently, the patient develops respiratory depression, requiring immediate airway management. The flaw inherent to this scenario was that the presenters' assumed that the participants would incorrectly overdose the patient with morphine.

During the conference, the participants did everything possible to avoid drug overdose: they used non-steroidal anti-inflammatory medications, ordered continued regional anesthesia, and ordered PCA pumps. Because the participants introduced appropriate safeguards, the presenters were forced to improvise a solution to keep the scenario running. The scenario participants received information that a novice nurse came and accidentally administered an additional dose of morphine, thus creating the rationale for the planned programmed outcome.

Multimedia as Prompts   Images and reports can include X-rays, radiology reports, 12-lead ECGs (static reports), ultrasound studies, CT scans, MRI, and others. Each new report, image, or document serves as *prompt* that will guide the participants during the scenario. The Parry Center used an interactive tablet-based system capable of presenting laboratory reports for blood work in real time. The system consists of the main computer (Mac or PC) and an iPad. It allows the facilitator/operator to manipulate the blood work results in real time and display the results for the participants on the iPad. This system was successfully piloted during a diabetic ketoacidosis (DKA) scenario for interprofessional education. Creative use of different simulation modalities as prompts can help expand a variety of simulated conditions for professional fields such as endocrinology, psychiatry, and neurology, who traditionally have not used simulation.

The reality is that three elements are needed to design a scenario:

1. Years of experience observing learners and the many possible good and poor interventions (or lack thereof) that are possible;
2. an imagination that answers the question "what if?" What if the learner/ participant
   • learner/participant: does _____?
   • does not do _____?
   • does nothing at all?
   • does something completely unanticipated?
3. Scenario design and programming must evolve with discovery of flaws and new opportunities.
   • Part of the discovery process includes
     ○ research of best practices, which change from time to time;
     ○ new protocols are developed, and
     ○ sometimes, new medications replace drugs that were previously appropriate.

The benefits of the SAO approach justify the time investment and include *consistency* in scenario facilitation and the ability to operate the simulator without needing a content expert to be present during the session.

STAGES OF SAO SCENARIO DEVELOPMENT

1. **Who are the participants?**

   As previously discussed, knowing who the intended participants are is critical to defining the learner's educational needs.

2. **What is the objective?**

   Based on the educational needs of the audience, a set of specific learning objectives must be developed, regardless of operational method (LIO/SAO).

3. **What teaching method will be selected?**

   Will the teaching method be a role modeling session with the instructor in the simulation room showing the learners the appropriate clinical procedures and guiding the participants during their performance? Will the teaching method be an interactive case based on the principles of *teaching by discovery* during which the participants will receive a short briefing and then allowed to obtain the rest of the relevant information to:

   - form a differential diagnosis,
   - initiate treatment,
   - evaluate the patient's response to treatment, and
   - redefine the differential diagnosis?

   For the scenario to be effective, each teaching method would require the scenario itself to be designed accordingly (Alinier, 2011).

4. **Create a flow chart of the scenario**

   Creating a paper-based or electronic flow chart of the scenario design. *This is the most important and potentially time-consuming part of scenario design.* All three first stages of the scenario design need to involve both clinical educators and SOSs.

5. **Automate the scenario**

   After the scenario design and implementation strategies are conceived, discussed, and documented, the programmer will *automate the scenario* as designed within the limits and capabilities of the simulator itself.

6. **Test the scenario**

   After the scenario is loaded onto the simulator and tested for programming errors, a test run should be conducted in order to evaluate how well interaction is between the participants and the simulator programming (Lioce et al., 2015, para. 224).

7. **Correct the scenario**

   Based on the results of the test run, both the scenario flow chart and the scenario facilitation method might need to be adjusted, and then the cycle repeats.

8. **Develop an evaluation instrument**

   During scenario development an evaluation instrument should be developed to enable the facilitator to determine if the learning objectives have been achieved. Debriefing is an important part of simulation. It allows learners to connect actions with patient outcomes and reduces faulty learning. Sometimes students may establish a faulty connection between an action and an unrelated coincident event.

For example, in a scenario in which the patient deteriorates and requires intubation, the patient vomits. The students might erroneously conclude that intubation provoked vomiting.

9. **Train facilitators and operations staff on how to use the scenario**

   When the scenario has been validated, clinical faculty and simulation operations staff must receive training on the correct facilitation of the scenario to ensure that the scenario is implemented consistently (standardized).

10. **Prepare the learners/participants**

    Whether through reading assignments, handouts, or lecture, and appropriate briefing, it is commonly accepted within the simulation community that such preparation would be beneficial to scenario participants. This will increase the probability that the participants will follow the correct path in the scenario and will derive greater satisfaction from simulation in general. Consider use of pre-scenario and post-scenario quizzes to assess the effectiveness of session. The benefit of this approach is that it allows improved assessment of participants' educational needs as well as measurement of the level of success of each session. At the same time, it has a potential for creating fixation and may give away the content of the scenario.

STUMBLING BLOCKS TO SUCCESSFUL SCENARIO IMPLEMENTATION

Old School Meets New School

No matter how good a design or programming method, the scenario can still fail if the operator/facilitator does not implement it appropriately. For example, an experienced clinician with limited exposure to simulation asks to facilitate a septic shock scenario. Rather than facilitate the scenario from a control room, he decides to be in the simulation room with the participants. When participants decide to start a dopamine infusion for hemodynamic support, the clinician interrupts the scenario, advises the participants they are to use norepinephrine rather than dopamine, and then lectures for 15 minutes on vasopressors. As a result, the participants are disengaged and have difficulty continuing the scenario. Unfortunately, too many scenarios fail because of the encroachment of traditional lecture styles into the simulation space or debriefing room. While some argue the merits of being present in the simulation space and even introducing instruction and new materials during the session, it is equally arguable that such actions are not appropriate for most high-fidelity simulation contexts (Horsley & Wambach, 2015, p. 6).

Insider Trading

Insider trading refers to those situations where learners share key elements of the scenario they just participated in with students who are about to do the same scenario.

Example   Suzie just finished a scenario where the patient was hyperglycemic and required 3 units of insulin based on the patient's blood glucose levels. She tells Jane who is about to participate, and Jane enters the scenario and immediately draws up insulin and administers it. Jane did not check the blood glucose results in the report, so did not calculate the dosage based on the glucose level. It was clear to the facilitator that Jane was privy to information about the scenario ahead of time, as the dosage was correct.

Design/Programming Solution   Program the scenario to include multiple blood glucose results varying from just above normal to very high. Randomly choose a different report for each scenario session and tell every student that each scenario will be different and they should NOT expect the same outcome as their peers. This will force the student to first learn what the report says, and then calculate the appropriate dosage.

Shell-Shocked

The learner is so nervous that they do nothing. The learner does not know what to do next and is afraid of doing the wrong thing.

Example   Sara enters the simulation room and stands at the patient's bedside. She begins to wring her hands and pace. After 10 minutes the facilitator is frustrated and ends the scenario session. The student is devastated and humiliated.

Design/Programming Solution   Have the "patient" or a confederate (perhaps, a family member comes in the room in such a situation) engage the learner in conversation. The simulator can say "Aren't you supposed to ask me some questions or something? That is what the last nurse did." This is known as a *prompt*. If the learner does not engage, the patient can begin to complain about why he is in the hospital—further trying to engage the learner. The patient can also introduce himself, and perhaps, remind the nurse about his allergies and his anxiety. A confederate could ask the learner "why are you here?" If the facilitator is the voice for the patient, he/she must be careful not to disclose too much information or accidentally misdirect the learner in the wrong direction. Ideally, vocals for the patient should be recorded and integrated into programming. This ensures that each learner has the same information as their peers. Granted, this is a lot more work, but standardization and automation help to better validate the scenario over time.

Tom-Foolery

Learners or others in the scenario may act unprofessionally and dismiss the scenario as a "fun" game.

Example   The learner enters the simulation room. He acts unprofessionally and makes unacceptable jokes.

Design/Programming Solution   The patient says, "I am sorry but I find the way you treat me disrespectful and unacceptable. I will file my complaint with the hospital administration." After this the session should be stopped, the student should take a break to refocus, and the session should start again from the beginning.

Loitering

Some learners have trouble "engaging" in the scenario for a variety of reasons. While the entire group of participants is involved with the patient, one or more learners do not participate.

Example   A group of six participants are all engaged with providing patient care, while the seventh participant, John, is just observing without any significant contribution to the care of the patient.

Design/Programming Solution   In this example, the group is too large. The optimal group size for high-fidelity simulation is three to four participants, at the most, five. If reducing the size of the group is not an option, then during the pre-scenario briefing, discuss the teamwork component of the session. The participants should also be instructed to select their team leader who will be responsible for delegating roles and responsibilities within the team.

Wandering Astray

Sometimes, learners start down a road during the scenario that was not anticipated, nor appropriate, to the focus of the scenario.

Example   A group of third-year medical students misinterprets the patient's cardiac rhythm and is unsuccessful in selecting the right treatment.

Design/Programming Solutions   Use prompts (previously described). If prompts are not achieving the goal, then have the group take a "time out." The facilitator can announce that the simulation session has been paused, and enters into the simulation room. She summarizes the clinical situation for the participants without giving direct recommendations. Often, a well-presented summary of the situation enables the students to recognize their mistake, and when the scenario resumes, begin to make satisfactory progress.

CONCLUSION

There are obvious and not so obvious benefits of designing and programming one's own scenarios:

* no license fees,
* freedom to use on multiple simulators,
* the scenario could be published on the PubMed and other peer-reviewed resources.
* improved standardization.

Programming one's own scenarios is an exciting and rewarding process, but it does not come without a challenge.

Writing a scenario requires *algorithmic* thinking and some programming skills. Even though programming scenarios is not the same as programming software, it still requires an understanding of basic programming concepts such as "if ... then" conditional statements, such as looping and nesting. The designer should be proficient in digital media manipulation to work with still images, video, and audio files. Proper documentation of the scenario programming features is still a continuing problem in simulation. Since there are multiple outcomes in the scenario that depend on the participants' actions, scenarios can unfold multiple ways. How does one document the scenario so that all outcomes are clearly described?

Scenario Programming and License Examinations

For years simulation has been considered for healthcare license examinations, however, this is yet to happen. There are two main challenges to this.

Unfortunately, the first challenge is simulation development cannot provide a standardized and consistent simulation experience (validated). Simulation operation is still very much operator-dependent, and thus open to human error. The second challenge is to provide the examiners with a valid and reliable evaluation tool. How can the evaluation tool be consistent if the simulation experience itself (in its current form) is inherently inconsistent? These two challenges create a vicious cycle that is not going to be resolved until substantial progress in simulation technology is achieved.

One of the ways to address this problem is to improve the automation and standardization of simulation programming software. The development of a standard simulation programming language that is manufacturer agnostic is needed. This language should be lean, irredundant, and flexible. All triggers, or events, and outcomes should be easy to program, record, and measure. The simulator should be able to directly, either through the manikin's sensors, or indirectly, through the operator's input, obtain information about the participant's actions and interpret it according to the programmed evaluation protocols (Slone & Lampotang, 2015, p. 190). The user interface of the scenario player should be minimalistic and should contain only relevant information. For example, if the scenario is SAO compliant, the operator does not need to see a live ECG on his or her control station. While running the simulator, it is enough to know the name of the patient's current cardiac rhythm. Only when the automation and standardization of patient simulation reaches certain levels will it be feasible to use high-fidelity simulation for high stakes license examinations. The authors of this chapter hope that their faith in automation and standardization in healthcare simulation will bring that day closer.

REFERENCES

Alinier, G. (2011, February 8). Developing high-fidelity health care simulation scenarios: A guide for educators and professionals. *Simulation & Gaming, 42*(1), 9–26.

Dieckmann, P., Lippert, A., Glavin, R., & Rall, M. (2010, August). When things do not go as expected: Scenario life savers. *Simulation in Healthcare, 5*(4), 219–225.

Gantt, L. (2012, November). Who's driving? the role and training of the human patient simulation operator. *CIN: Computers, Informatics, Nursing, 30,* 579–586.

Horsley, T. L., & Wambach, K. (2015). Anxiety, self-confidence, and clinical performance during a clinical simulation experience. *Clinical Simulation in Nursing, 11*(1), 4–10.

Lioce, L., Meakim, C. H., Fey, M. K., Chmil, J. V., Mariani, B., & Alinier, G. (2015). Standards of best practice: Simulation standard IX: design. *Clinical Simulation in Nursing, 11*(6), 309–315.

Slone, F. L., & Lampotang, S. (2015). Mannequins: terminology, selection, and usage. In J. C. Palaganas, J. C. Maxworthy, C. A. Epps, & M. E. Mancini (Eds.), *Defining excellence in simulation programs* (pp. 183–198). Hong Kong: Wolters Kluwer.

11

SIMULATION OPERATIONS SPECIALISTS JOB DESCRIPTIONS COMPOSITION, NEGOTIATION, AND PROCESSES

LAURA T. GANTT

East Carolina University College of Nursing, Greenville, NC, USA

A frequently asked question for online simulation networking sites pertains to what job title to give to the simulation technologists on the operations team. The following is an incomplete list of what an individual who supports simulation technology may be called:

- Simulation specialist
- Simulation technician or technologist
- Simulation technology specialist
- Simulation lab assistant
- Operations specialist
- Education and technology specialist
- Simulation educator.

The dilemma of what title to give this professional group stems from a variety of issues. First, the role of the simulation operations specialist (SOS) has been in constant evolution as the use of simulation in healthcare has continued to expand.

Healthcare Simulation: A Guide for Operations Specialists, First Edition.
Edited by Laura T. Gantt and H. Michael Young.
© 2016 John Wiley & Sons, Inc. Published 2016 by John Wiley & Sons, Inc.

Education and training that once included static manikins and task trainers now include full body simulators and virtual reality. As recently as 10 years ago, all simulation-related roles may have been handled by one or two people, typically clinicians or educators, even in large centers. In some centers, it may still be the case that multiple functions are being handled by very few people; for some, this system may work well. However, other centers have recognized the need for a dedicated SOS whose job is to oversee the technology functions of the overall simulation enterprise. Within this chapter the SOS will be referred to as the operations specialist. Regardless of what job title is eventually assigned to the SOS, there is a procedure for writing a job description or choosing a pre-existing one for the position. The purpose of this chapter is to describe this process.

WRITING A NEW JOB DESCRIPTION

For the purpose of this chapter, a position description is defined as *the information which may be posted about a particular job, as well as the associated evaluation for the position.* A position description may appear to be short in and of itself (see Appendix 2 for a position description for a technology support technician). However, since employees must be evaluated on their performance at the end of a specified amount of time, it may work best to work backward. Begin the job description development process by envisioning objective measures of performance for the particular job for which the overall description needs to be written.

The sample evaluation for a technology support technician included in Appendix 2 may be a useful reference. Though they may vary from one organization to another, most performance evaluations for any given job description will include three or four major sections:

1. *Core values*

   The first section describes core values of the organization or overarching expectations of employee behavior and conduct. Within an organization, this section should look much the same for every job description or performance evaluation.

2. *Key responsibilities*

   The second section outlines key responsibilities or job duties on which the employee will be evaluated. This section tends to be the largest part of the evaluation, as well as the section from which the job description may be drawn.

3. *Competency or functional assessment*

   A third area may be competency assessment, which defines the level at which an employee performs key responsibilities. For example, a new employee and an employee with 10 years of experience function at different competency levels, though both may perform within acceptable ranges for the competency level determined by their job description. Not all job descriptions or performance evaluations contain this category.

4. *Management or leadership responsibilities*

Fourth and finally, many job descriptions also contain supervisory, human resource management, or leadership components, which may be rated or deemed not applicable for a given employee.

THE FIRST STEP: WHAT WILL THE SOS DO?

Creating a new job description begins with determining the desired job functions. It may be possible to obtain job descriptions from simulation organization websites or from colleagues who already have an operations specialist or similar role in their departments. Job descriptions from other organizations provide a place to start and help generate ideas, even if they turn out not to have all of the desired components. Operations specialist job descriptions may vary somewhat by setting; one example from an academic setting (technology support specialist) and one from a clinical setting (simulation specialist) are included in Appendix 2.

If no previously created operations specialist position descriptions are available, then there are a few ways to generate principal job duties. Many organizations have a prescribed position description template; this should be located before beginning the work of task analysis and may be most commonly found in human resources departments or from persons in supervisory positions.

A task or job analysis involves an extensive study of a specific position using data from several sources. If there is a person who is already doing part of the work for which a new position description is being prepared, it is well worth having that person involved in ensuring that all the necessary job functions are included. Other members of the simulation team should also be able to name at least some of the job duties for the proposed position description. A job description that makes its way between different personnel in a simulation center during its development allows for multiple viewpoints that increase team acceptance of the position over the long term.

Once the key responsibilities of the position have been outlined, it should become clear whether it will take an average person a full workweek to do the job versus some part of the week. One full-time equivalent means that the job duties take roughly 40 hours/week to complete. After assigning percentages of time spent or allotted to each key job duty in a position description, the total of the percentages should equal 100.

Job specifications or requirements that support the performance of key responsibilities must also be determined. Job specifications describe the extent of specific skills, effort, and responsibilities required of the person in the position (Fallon & McConnell, 2014). In the case of the SOS, job specifications may include an instructional technology degree or certifications in a healthcare-related field. The Society for Simulation in Healthcare (SSH) has developed a certification exam for healthcare simulation operations specialists (CHSOS) that includes an examination blueprint. The blueprint outlines knowledge that operations specialists should have, which could assist in writing of job descriptions and evaluations.

Job specifications should also include licensure or educational requirements that may be tied to compensation, which must be kept in mind if there is a certain amount of funding tied to the position. For example, if a position is budgeted for a salary of no more than \$50,000 per year, the job requirements may be different than if the salary can be adjusted according to qualifications. Funding level for a position may also affect whether supervisory functions are part of the position description, since oversight of other personnel justifies and necessitates a higher salary. Unfortunately, at times, the job description must be written to fit the funds allotted to a position, rather than the other way around.

Many organizations expect their employees to exhibit and support certain core values, as mentioned previously, such as integrity and a respect for diversity. All employees will receive ratings on how well they demonstrate adherence to these organizational norms.

In light of the fact that widespread use of simulation in healthcare has occurred relatively recently, there may be few available candidates for an SOS position. When writing the position description, the author must give thought to who might have the closest type of related experience or educational preparation. Previous training or experience in simulation is the exception, rather than the rule, when recruiting for almost any position in a healthcare simulation center.

EXISTING JOB DESCRIPTIONS AND CLASSIFICATIONS

In many organizations, it is not possible to assign a new job title and a corresponding position description. Instead, when hiring a new employee, candidates apply for a job based on an *existing* job description. In larger institutions, similar job titles and position descriptions are grouped to ensure salary equity. Hence, it may be the case that there are technology-related job descriptions in a job class that provide the basis for all such positions. For example, in the aforementioned job descriptions in Appendix 2, the technology support technician position most closely resembles the job functions required of the beginning operations specialist within that organization. The advantage of this way of managing job descriptions is that it takes a lot of the guesswork out of getting a position description written and funded at an appropriate level; funding, in this case, refers to the salary and benefits for the person hired into a particular position. The downside of this approach is that a position like SOS may not fit well with any existing job descriptions that the organization has already written. When one looks closely at the technology support technician position, for example, it can be seen that the job description seems non-specific that translation will be required to determine how the SOS will carry out the job functions within the simulation center.

The good news is that it is possible to have both *official* and *functional* job descriptions for any position. The *official* job description reflects those job components that the organization has agreed should be common to every employee within a certain job class. The *functional* or "working" description may be more specific to the day-to-day work that the employee does within a department.

To take the example of the employee within a department who functions as an SOS, his official job description may be technical support technician, as is the description for any number of employees across the organization. In this case, the official description focuses on the technical knowledge and other skill sets required by the job. However, this employee's functional or working job description includes the specifics of that same knowledge base as it relates to healthcare simulation, simulators, and operations within the learning environment. The functional job description may be maintained with or separately from the official position description, which makes it difficult, in some cases, to get copies of both. The functional parts of the job become a title used within the organization. This is how the employee officially titled as the technology support technician becomes known as the simulation specialist.

A few words of caution must be included here about the alignment of official and functional job descriptions. If the difference between official and functional job descriptions is too great, it will be difficult to evaluate employee performance. Performance evaluations are generally tied to *official* job descriptions. This necessitates the best possible fit between more than one position description used to define the work of any individual or group of employees. Another problem arises from trying to include too many types of job functions within one position description, especially when some of the responsibilities are really part of a completely different position description.

NEGOTIATING INTERNAL AND EXTERNAL PROCESSES TO GET THE JOB DESCRIPTION APPROVED AND FILLED

The person charged with creating a new position description has a great deal of negotiating to do. In truth, the new position must be supported by key people in the organization from its inception. Regardless of whether there is an existing job description or a new one is created, the timeline for task analysis, composition of the document, and getting necessary approvals can be a long one. This process will go more smoothly when those who grant approvals for positions are well-informed about the position. It is not unusual for the draft job description to travel between its author and human resources departments several times before it moves from the description phase to a determination of compensation and benefits. The working draft may be forwarded to management staff, usually several people, who will grant separate approvals to it. Realistically, from the time a new position is conceived until the time the position is ready for posting and advertising can take at least 6 months.

Once the SOS position makes it to the point where it is posted, figuring out how to advertise it can prove challenging. There is no clear choice of places to publicize this type of position. Obviously, if there is a person within an organization who is qualified for and capable of fulfilling the job requirements, then that employee can be considered after organizational human resource rules are followed. For example, most institutions will require interviewing more than one candidate, even if one or more applicants are internal applicants. If there are no such persons within the organization, then local, regional, and national advertising can be considered using job or organizational website postings or print media, based on the size and type of the desired applicant pool. In academic environments or in organizations near colleges and universities, new graduates with specified degrees may be recruited. If other job searches are going on with the institution, one job search may yield suitable candidates for other searches as well. Finally, there is a lot to be said for word of mouth in recruiting applicants for positions. Colleagues in other health science departments may know qualified applicants looking for job opportunities.

There are a few potentially unique considerations for the interviewing of SOSs. It can be hard for most applicants to envision what goes on in a simulation lab, much less understand what their role in the lab might be. Interview processes for simulation lab staff may need to include a lab or facility tour. Some organizations also plan on a two-stage interview process in which the applicants observe activities in the simulation lab and spend some time interacting with other staff in the area; this enables both applicant and organization a chance to get to know one another better.

CONCLUSION

Since simulation activities are not facilitated by any one person in isolation, the communication skills of the SOS are of significant importance. Simulation design and implementation may involve any combination of faculty, staff, learners, or interprofessional teams. The design of the position description should focus on the set of skills that candidate who is selected must have to function within the simulation environment. The individual tasked with writing the job description and negotiating it toward fulfillment must be able to articulate and describe a job that is both new and quickly evolving as roles within the field of simulation expand. For creative approaches in developing SOS job descriptions, the reader is also referred to Chapter 8.

REFERENCE

Fallon, L. F., & McConnell, C. R. (2014). *Human resource management in health care: Principles and Practice* (2nd ed., pp. 115–123). Burlington, MA: Jones & Bartlett Learning.

12

SIMULATION RESEARCH AND THE ROLE OF THE SIMULATION OPERATIONS SPECIALIST

GENE W. HOBBS

University of North Carolina, Chapel Hill, NC, USA

INTRODUCTION

One of the most important roles of the simulation operations specialist (SOS, OS) is the orchestration of a unique, effective educational experience. The SOS does this by participating in all aspects of the day-to-day operations of the simulation center, from developing simulation goals and objectives, to implementing the scenarios or cases with learners, to the many tasks that go on behind the scenes. Setting up equipment, planning resources, and creative problem-solving are only a few of the talents the SOS brings to the enterprise. The SOS is also accountable for the budget to accomplish these tasks in a safe and procedurally sound manner. Often this also includes securing funding for the next cycle or year of training. In many cases, the SOS may be the primary person recruiting both new faculty and learners to join in simulation opportunities.

Each of these talents described above requires special attention to detail. In 1992, the Association of Clinical Research Professionals (ACRP) offered the first Certified Clinical Research Coordinator (CCRC) exams (Education Portal, 2015). The skills that operations specialists utilize on a daily basis to achieve educational outcomes are similar to the competencies the ACRP requires of clinical research coordinators in accomplishing research outcomes.

Healthcare Simulation: A Guide for Operations Specialists, First Edition.
Edited by Laura T. Gantt and H. Michael Young.
© 2016 John Wiley & Sons, Inc. Published 2016 by John Wiley & Sons, Inc.

SIMULATION OPERATIONS SPECIALISTS AS A RESOURCE

Principal investigators (PI) rely on clinical research coordinators to help them plan, budget, test protocols, and execute research studies. PIs for simulation-based research consult SOSs for these same duties, so it is important for the SOS to understand research roles as well.

Nobody knows the simulation environment better than the SOS does. An SOS will know what equipment will be available, what additional resources can be brought to bear, and what will work or not work within a specific simulation center. The SOS also knows how to safely operate the equipment utilized within the simulation environment.

Since clinical equipment in simulation labs may be fully functional while other equipment such as defibrillators may be modified for simulation purposes, the SOS serves a critical role in safety protocol development. The welfare of simulation research subjects and study personnel is one of the most important duties of an SOS, regardless of the plan for any given day.

DATA COLLECTION AND INTEGRITY

In light of recent public exposure of potential unethical practices by PIs in conducting and publishing their research, and the subsequent retraction of articles (Katavic, 2014), specialists serve as a valuable resource in the data collection and integrity chain.

The 2009 case of Anil Potti, a cancer researcher at Duke University, received international attention when a paper was published showing that data from a study by Dr. Potti was mislabeled and mismatched (Anonymous, 2011; Nelson, 2011). While some questions exist that these errors were the result of malicious tampering, the case emphasizes the need for researchers to protect against any potential impropriety. If a researcher has any potential proprietary interest in the results of an experiment, operations specialists can serve as an additional cross-check to prevent conflicts of interest.

Operations specialists can protect raw data to ensure that no opportunity for tampering exists between collection and statistical analysis. Recently, journal editors have begun to request analysis by third party statisticians, which means that proper handling of raw data has become even more critical. Operations specialists in the field must ensure that ethical practices are not called into question since they may be co-investigators on grants and may be subject to the same bias as other team members.

Research subjects are at potential risk of exposure of personal data to others outside the research team. Many research studies include collection of subject interactions or tasks that are collected on video. Subjects could experience short- or long-term educational or professional harm if these videos were to be released publicly. The SOS understands available opportunities for data collection and security. This allows the operations specialist to best advise the primary investigators as they devise their protocols.

Security and Protection

The ACRP provides recommendations for the security and protection of data within their standards and certification and constantly updates their members on protocols and laws that may impact them.

Healthcare simulation team members who are either hospital-based or have some interactions with academic healthcare systems are familiar with requirements imposed by the Health Insurance Portability and Accountability Act (HIPAA) and Family Educational Rights and Privacy Act (FERPA). Operations specialists also need to make sure other members of the research team, like standardized patients or educational facilitators, are familiar with requirements of the law (Messina, Smith, & Hobbs, 2015). This can be especially important if the study will happen *in situ* and incidental contact with patients and care providers and can occur.

Something that may be new to SOSs moving into research is the world of Institutional Review Boards (IRB) established by the federal government to ensure that research subjects are protected. An example can be found in the Tuskegee Syphilis Study that ran from 1932 to 1972 by the U.S. Public Health Service. The study tracked the natural progression of syphilis in untreated African-American males who believed they were receiving free healthcare. The men recruited for the study were sharecroppers who were provided access to medical care, meals, and free burial to incentivize them to participate. None of the men were informed of their syphilis diagnosis. Even after penicillin was recognized as a proven treatment for the disease in 1947, the men remained untreated. The National Research Act of 1974 was passed to address disconnects between human rights and scientific research and established guidelines for human subjects research, as well as oversight and regulation of human trials. As a result of this Act, subjects must be informed of risks, diagnoses must be communicated, and test results must be reported.

The National Research Act of 1974 was followed by the Belmont Report in 1978. The report identified three core principles and three primary areas of application. The principles of respect for persons, beneficence, and justice ensure that researchers are truthful with no deception, "do no harm" with respect to risk versus benefits to the subjects, and research is conducted fairly.

Because of the risk of bias, PIs may not always be able to see all the data they collect. In a study performed by the chapter author, one of the PIs was only able to score video of his colleagues and not those of anesthesia residents he might supervise clinically in the future (Segall, Taekman, Mark, Hobbs, & Wright, 2007; Wright, Segall, Mark, Hobbs, & Taekman, 2007). The IRB at the institution was concerned that poor responses or decisions by the resident in the trial could bias the researcher's future clinical assessments when they work together.

In facilitating research studies, the operations specialist can also serve an essential role in the experimental design. "Blinding" is a method to increase the accuracy of data collected by ensuring that researchers, participants, and other staff do not influence the data being collected. It is an important part of research because it prevents intentional or unconscious bias. While operating simulators, the SOS has the ability to blind both the subject and the PI or researcher from knowing exactly which test state is being performed; blinding both subject and researcher is called double blinding. This can have a significant impact on the validity of an experiment.

Another example of how specialists can protect a study is by facilitating order balancing or counterbalancing for the protocol when repeated measures are needed. The order in which events are tested can confound study variables and significantly impact results. For example, if a group of subjects is tested on two items in the same order for each, the researcher may not know what information the subjects gathered as a result of the ordering. The subjects could be learning in the first exposure and applying that knowledge to the second exposure and therefore impacting the results. The most common way to control this is by random selection of events (randomized order). In large studies, it is very important that randomized order be followed, but also just as important that counterbalancing occurs when needed (University of North Carolina at Chapel Hill, Psychology Department, 2008).

Counterbalancing is another way of reducing the impact of participant errors by breaking the subjects into groups and giving the groups a different order. In the research design, counterbalancing controls for the order of treatments or educational interventions to prevent researchers from drawing incorrect conclusions about the impact of their intervention. For example, if the plan is to teach something two ways, such as using virtual (V) and mannequin (M) simulation methods, the class would be split into groups. Then the training would be provided to half the groups in VM order and the other half in MV order. This makes the variance a separate order effect which makes for a more powerful experimental design.

Studies may require multiple PIs to make decisions; researchers may be paying attention to so many moving parts that they miss errors related to the order of variables in the experiment. Lack of careful oversight can lead to issues with statistics and eventually publication. The specialist is likely to be present for each experimental condition. This unique view of the protocol as it progresses allows the operations specialist to interact with the PIs to prevent errors.

RESEARCH METHODS AND PROJECT EXAMPLES

Throughout this book, there are many types of simulations, training, and outcomes discussed. The same can be said of the types of research encompassed by simulation. In this section, there are several examples of how simulation is applied to address research needs.

Models and Data Simulations

Though many people think of the models used in simulations as a part of the tool, they can also be powerful for research and education all by themselves. Mathematical models exist in medicine to explain phenomena like drug uptake and elimination, physiological responses to various stimuli, and equipment operations.

In 2007, the Rubicon Foundation, Inc. began their Decompression Application Risk Assessment (DARA) project (Rubicon Foundation, 2011). The goal of this project was to assess the risk that divers would be undertaking when following guidelines presented to them by commercially available software. This project utilized simulations for these profiles in conjunction with a risk assessment tool designed by Dr. Wayne Gerth for the U.S. Navy. These model-driven simulations have provided real-life guidance in the performance of individual activities which may significantly impact safety.

This chapter's author, in his role as an SOS, was able to assist Dr. Laurens Howle at Duke University in the development of a tool to format the dive profile information, such as time and depth. Once the tool was tested, the SOS was able to translate profile information into the type of inputs required by the models for the risk assessment.

In October of 2014, BioGears was released by a team headed by investigator Jerry Heneghan at Applied Research Associates. BioGears is a series of open source physiology and pharmacology models that allow users to test drugs and interventions, or learn more about these, without the risk to patients. The software works in a similar way to models imbedded into simulation mannequin programming, but does not require the expensive hardware or interfaces to access the results. The BioGears development team utilized operations specialists for developing the initial scenarios released with the software. Operations specialists are now validating new models and developing additional cases to more fully utilize this innovative resource.

Almost every new anesthesia provider comes across the Virtual Anesthesia Machine (VAM) developed by team lead Dr. Sem Lampotang at the University of Florida. Dr. Lampotang developed and tested the VAM model for training providers on the use of anesthetic gasses and equipment operations to improve learning of a complex piece of medical equipment (Lampotang, Lizdas, & Gravenstein, 2006). Dr. Lampotang's team of operations specialists developed and tested not only the accuracy of the VAM model, but also the educational value this form of transparent reality offers learners (Fischler, Kaschub, Lizdas, & Lampotang, 2008). Simulation operations specialists offer valuable expertise to the development of these projects by ensuring that they mimic reality as closely as possible and that medical content is as accurate as feasible. Once projects are underway, the SOS plays a key role in data collection and, in many cases, the data analysis. Specialists on this team also utilized the VAM to evaluate the utility of checklists used by anesthesia providers for daily equipment checks (Lampotang, Moon, Lizdas, Feldman, & Zhang, 2005).

Human Factors Engineering

The aviation community has utilized simulators to test new equipment and procedures for decades. Human factors engineers are now evaluating medical equipment, procedures, and task analytic activities within simulation environments in order to prevent risk to actual patients (Wright & Taekman, 2003).

Medical Equipment Testing

SOSs can also assist with the development of scenarios designed to evaluate user interfaces and menu structure for machines such as infusion pumps. The operations specialist may design scenarios that require nurses to make adjustments to drug doses, add infusions, and disconnect or reconnect the patient while taking care of other potentially distracting clinical tasks like monitor alarms or calls from other patients.

The SOS can play an equally important role on clinical equipment committees to assist with health system decisions on the purchase of new equipment and subsequent staff training in the clinical environment. Basic usability studies such as this one can be extremely helpful in making decisions that can limit latent errors in equipment designs and also help identify potential user mistakes.

Similarly, the SOS can help with departmental and system wide quality improvement (QI) research projects. By recreating situations where errors have occurred, the specialist can assist with root cause analysis research, as well as implementation of the engineering or training solutions to prevent these problems in the future. For example, consider the high profile cases of patients who have received blood administration of the wrong type. By re-enacting the cases in the simulation environment, identifying where the problems occurred can lead to changes that may prevent future such errors.

Another problem often facing hospital leadership is that of staffing requirements. Teamwork trials have helped identify staffing deficiencies during which team members were unable to assist each other with ease in emergencies. As the trials continued, other problems within the system began to further impede care if a second event requiring more than just normal staffing for patient situations occurred. These findings can lead to changes in on-call and on-site staff requirements and help with budget justifications for the hiring of additional staff.

Dr. Noa Segall at Duke University completed a study looking at cardiac telemetry workload and staffing. The hospital sought to change the number of patient beds each telemetry technician would be required to monitor during a shift. To complete this study, the research team had to recreate their normal workload of the telemetry technicians, as well as incorporate adverse events into the recorded data stream (Segall et al., 2015).

The operations specialist for this study made the recordings needed and assisted the team in developing a method for the fake adverse event to occur without an obvious change in the recording. They then ensured that the data streams had been properly de-identified and set up the mock telemetry lab with recording equipment to capture the study tasks. Similar needs existed for the Trinity Health study; the operations specialists also mocked up various work environments for the evaluations. They modified their center to have local, remote, and hybrid monitoring stations by building the work environment and adding the equipment normally used in these conditions (Wright et al., 2014). Further study into this topic performed by Trinity Health resulted in suggestions on how quality monitoring could be accomplished for varying environmental constraints (Wright et al., 2014).

Dr. Segall was also asked by her hospital to do an analysis of common tasks performed on the online patient portal. For this study, the operations specialist was able to serve as a test subject, as well as assist in setting up a portable recording solution for the capture of the usage data. The subjects recruited for this trial were volunteer patients being seen at a clinic associated with the hospital system. The changes suggested by the research team led to changes in the user experience and improved access to their medical records and test results.

When researching the roles of individuals and how they function within their work environment, SOSs can also assist with research on complex tasks and teamwork. Design and execution of large studies requires utilization of the specialist's skills as an innovator, networker, collaborator, operator, and facilitator. Depending on the tasks and or work being observed, skills as an artist, producer, director, and conductor may also be required. As the complexity of a task or procedure grows, increased personnel requirements can necessitate that the SOS take on a larger role in development and management of the project.

Following a 2009 evaluation of tasks involved in sedation by anesthesiologists and gastroenterologists for patients undergoing upper gastrointestinal (GI) endoscopy at the VA Medical Center in Durham NC, a training program was developed with the intention of increasing the safety for this patient population (Schroeder, Barbeito, Segall, & Mark, 2009). In developing the cases that would be used for this training, the SOS was consulted to help script the scenario and prepare the training team for simulation operations *in situ*. Since the cases occurred in a room with the training team and clinicians in close proximity, the SOS developed a system for nonverbal communication to facilitate a more personalized scenario given the interactions of the learner with the simulated patient. This training program was eventually published by the team and released as a toolkit for moderate sedation training (VA National Center for Patient Safety, 2015). Specialists continue to assist the monitoring desired outcomes following the training interventions.

In 2012, the Durham VA published a literature review on perioperative handovers (Segall et al., 2012). This was the first step in a much larger project to improve patient safety during this complex procedure of making sure that care teams communicate all pertinent information to the team that is receiving the patient.

This study showed how an SOS is a valuable part of new projects, starting from the early literature review to development of training protocols for quality improvement and patient safety in later phases of research and education. By being a part of the team early in the development process, operations specialists are able to provide guidance to the team to meet goals that can be accomplished within the program constraints of time, equipment, and personnel.

The Standardized Assessment for Evaluation of Team Skills (SAFE-TeamS) project was published in 2013 by researchers from Trinity Health, Duke University, and the North Carolina Hospital Association (Wright et al., 2013). This project utilized actors as members of the healthcare team to place medical and nursing students into challenging situations that required their use of "ideal behaviors associated with assistance, conflict resolution, communication, assertion, and situation assessment."

For this study, the operations specialist was able to provide context for development of the simulations, recruited and trained the actors for the varied roles portrayed, and ensured that all props and equipment was assembled for the scenarios. The specialist was also involved in data management and de-identification of the pre- versus post-training conditions for the clinical monitors scoring the interactions so that the monitors would not be biased to which condition they were scoring.

A pediatric resident training research project for the implementation of TeamSTEPPS in critical care environments was conducted by the University of North

Carolina. This project utilized pre- and post-training communication evaluations with the Teamwork Evaluation of Non-Technical Skills (TENTS) training tool.

Specialists in this project were able to provide training to the raters before the trial began. A significant amount of data management was required to ensure that raters were blinded to the condition under evaluation and to provide on-demand access to the videos to ensure compliance with IRB requirements.

Real and Virtual Environments

In 2010, the Duke Department of Obstetrics, guided by Dr. Evelyn Lockhart in Transfusion Services, addressed the need to develop an interdisciplinary protocol for the treatment of postpartum hemorrhage (Lockhart, 2014). The team began by creating a simulation case to evaluate existing procedures utilized by their teams. Data was collected on various time sensitive events starting with the length of time it took for the team to begin arriving at the bedside. From there, the team established a protocol and training schedule to ensure all staff was in a constant state of readiness (Lockhart, Allen, Gunatilake, Hobbs, & Taekman, 2012).

After the protocol had been established *in situ* with mannequins, efforts began to build a virtual environment for this case funded by a grant to Dr. Barbara Turner from the Health Resources and Services Administration (Lockhart et al., 2013). The virtual environment was then utilized by South Australia for team training to improve healthcare communication for their region (South Australia. Department of Health. Safety and Quality Unit, 2014). Most recently, the team evaluated the use of this virtual environment for training staff in Uganda where a high maternal mortality rate could be addressed with this tool (Duke University School of Medicine, Duke Anesthesiology, 2014).

From the initial training sessions that the Duke obstetrics team performed *in situ*, until the most recent distance education efforts, the scenarios, materials, and curricula were impacted by many operations specialists. The importance of a specialist to this project was most apparent in making the situation seem realistic and in capturing the opportunities for improvement given the limited resources available for the training and research. All the skills of an innovator were used in finding solutions to limitations within the environments. The skills of a networker were essential to build relationships with clinicians to get to a final product. The talents of a collaborator were needed in building teams for interdisciplinary efforts. The abilities of an operator were required to execute the simulations. The gifts of a facilitator were brought to bear in training sessions to get clinicians through the technological challenges.

Dr. William McIvor and a team of anesthesia physicians and researchers published preliminary data evaluating the effectiveness of simulations performed for Maintenance of Certification for Anesthesiologists (MOCA®) recertification in 2012. The MOCA® research team utilized specialists in planning the trials from the initial scenario scripting and testing to learner data gathering and analysis. This ongoing study showed that the first 583 participants viewed the process as an experiential learning opportunity and that it was effective in promoting practice improvement (McIvor, Burden, Weinger, & Steadman, 2012). In the first 2 years the American

Society of Anesthesiologists reported that 98% of all participants felt the training was relevant to their practice (Steadman, Berry, Coursin, & Andrews, 2013).

Educational and Curriculum

The best way to apply lessons learned in all research performed by simulation teams is by incorporating the tools and findings from the research environment to educational needs through the curriculum.

Even though recent work has increased its acceptance, simulation as a whole still faces an uphill battle for recognition as a valuable education and safety tool. The reasons for this may range from administrators who do not see the need to spend money when they feel it does not impact their health system's bottom line to the attitudes of highly qualified clinicians in being "trained" more on concepts they do not see the need for. In educational terms, we have not always done a good job conveying the principle of effect to our communities.

The 2014 release of the National Council of State Boards of Nursing (NCSBN) simulation study has made a significant impact on acceptance of simulation as a valid tool for providing expertise to clinicians (National Council of State Boards of Nursing (NCSBN), 2014a).

These researchers replaced clinical hours with simulation experiences. They were able to show that there was no significant difference in board test scores between the students that had more live patients and those that had more simulator experiences (National Council of State Boards of Nursing (NCSBN), 2014b). The NCSBN teams accomplished this project with assistance from many specialists. These specialists were responsible for designing and implementation of the cases as well as data collection.

A 2010 publication of a research project evaluating learning styles was funded by Glaxo Smith Kline (GSK). The GSK project evaluated teaching of different concepts to maximize how TeamSTEPPS principles are learned and subsequent retention of that knowledge (Hobgood et al., 2010). For this project, a team of operations specialists were used to set-up and coordinate the huge groups of medical and nursing students through their cases. A study that manages 438 research subjects from two universities and is conducted over a 1-day period with four experimental conditions would be impossible without specialists that are able to adapt to a new environment, equipment, and manage their own teams for efficient operations.

The simulation team in the Duke University anesthesia department performed a smaller study evaluating live mannequin-based simulations, virtual environments, and didactic training. This team found that high-fidelity simulation was desirable, but required a higher instructor to trainee ratio that the virtual environment (Segall et al., 2011).

In a 2014 study from the National University of Singapore and the University of Newcastle looking at skills degradation, both methods were shown to be effective for skills retention but neither showed a real advantage over the other (Liaw, Chan, Chen, Hooi, & Siau, 2014).

CONCLUSION

The unique skills and perspective brought to the research team by the SOS adds tremendous value to both experimental design and execution. Research studies do not always need to be about research itself. They can also serve as a vehicle for development and promotion of employees or even provide continued medical education to those that participate.

ACKNOWLEDGMENTS

Melanie Wright, PhD; Noa Segall, PhD; Jerry Heneghan; Heather Frederick, MD; Benny Joyner, MD, MPH; Becky Hobbs, RN, MSN; Virginia Carden, MLS.

REFERENCES

Anonymous. (2011). Science and technology: An array of errors; misconduct in science. *The Economist, 400*(8750), 91–92.

Duke University School of Medicine, Duke Anesthesiology. (2014). Recent research grants. *Duke Anesthesiology*. Retrieved from http://anesthesiology.duke.edu/?p=828501

Education Portal. (2015). Certified Clinical Research Coordinator (CCRC) exams. *Clinical research coordinator certification program overviews*. Retrieved from http://education-portal. com/clinical_research_coordinator_certification.html

Fischler, I. S., Kaschub, C. E., Lizdas, D. E., & Lampotang, S. (2008). Understanding of anesthesia machine function is enhanced with a transparent reality simulation. *Simulation in Healthcare, 3*(1), 26–32. doi:10.1097/SIH.0b013e31816366d3

Hobgood, C., Sherwood, G., Frush, K., Hollar, D., Maynard, L., Foster, B., ... Taekman, J. (2010). Teamwork training with nursing and medical students: Does the method matter? Results of an interinstitutional, interdisciplinary collaboration. *Quality Safety in Health Care, 19*(6), e25. doi:10.1136/qshc.2008.031732

Katavic, V. (2014). Retractions of scientific publications: Responsibility and accountability. *Biochemical Medica: Casopis Hrvatskoga Drustva Medicinskih Biokemicara, 24*(2), 217–222. doi:10.11613/bm.2014.024

Lampotang, S., Lizdas, D. E., & Gravenstein, N. (2006). Transparent reality: A simulation based on interactive dynamic graphical models emphasizing visualization. *Educational Technology, 46*(6), 55–59.

Lampotang, S., Moon, S., Lizdas, D. E., Feldman, J. M., & Zhang, R. V. (2005). Anesthesia machine pre-use check survey—Preliminary results. *Anesthesiology, 103*(Suppl), A1195.

Liaw, S. Y., Chan, S. W., Chen, F. G., Hooi, S. C., & Siau, C. (2014). *Comparison of virtual patient simulation with mannequin-based simulation for improving clinical performances in assessing and managing clinical deterioration: Randomized controlled trial. Journal of Medical Internet Research, 16*(9), e214. doi:10.2196/jmir.3322

Lockhart, E. (2014). Transfusion management of obstetric hemorrhage. *The Global Library of Women's Medicine*. Retrieved from https://www.glowm.com/pdf/PPH_2nd_edn_Chap-04.pdf

Lockhart, E., Allen, T., Gunatilake, R., Hobbs, G., & Taekman, J. M. (2012, January 31). *Use of human simulation for the development of a multidisciplinary obstetric massive transfusion protocol.* Paper presented at the 12th International Meeting on Simulation in Healthcare, San Diego, CA.

Lockhart, E., Allen, T., Steele, M., Bonifacio, A., Hobbs, G., & Taekman, J. M. (2013). Board 525—Technology innovations abstract: Development of a multiplayer virtual-reality obstetric hemorrhage simulation program (Submission #747). *Simulation in Healthcare, 8*(6), 621.

McIvor, W., Burden, A., Weinger, M. B., & Steadman, R. (2012). Simulation for maintenance of certification in anesthesiology: The first two years. *Journal of Continuing Education in the Health Professions, 32*(4), 236–242. doi:10.1002/chp.21151

Messina, J., Smith, K., & Hobbs, G. W. (2015, June). From the skills center to the clinic: Preparing SPs for in situ simulations. *Association of Standardized Patient Educators Annual Scientific Meeting.* Denver, CO.

National Council of State Boards of Nursing (NCSBN). (2014a). The NCSBN national simulation study: A longitudinal, randomized, controlled study replacing clinical hours with simulation in prelicensure nursing education. *Journal of Nursing Regulation, 5*(2 Suppl), S4–64.

National Council of State Boards of Nursing (NCSBN). (2014b, August 21). NCSBN Releases Results of National Simulation Study. *NCSBN News Releases.* Retrieved from https://www.ncsbn.org/5507.htm

Nelson, R. (2011). Dr. Potti and Duke University sued over faulty research. *Medscape Medical News.* Retrieved from http://www.medscape.com/viewarticle/749577

Rubicon Foundation. (2011). Decompression application risk assessment. *Rubicon Foundation Projects.* Retrieved from http://rubicon-foundation.org/Projects/decompression-application-risk-assessment/

Schroeder, R. A., Barbeito, A., Segall, N., & Mark, J. B. (2009). A992: Sedation for upper GI rndoscopy: Practice patterns of anesthesiologists and gastroenterologists. *ASA Abstracts.* Retrieved from http://www.asaabstracts.com/strands/asaabstracts/abstract.htm;jsessionid=D97BD920058BFF7EC6B7F9EE636F3547?year=2009&index=15&absnum=1348

Segall, N., Bonifacio, A. S., Schroeder, R. A., Barbeito, A., Rogers, D., Thornlow, D. K., … Mark, J. B. (2012). Can we make postoperative patient handovers safer? A systematic review of the literature. *Anesthesia and Analgesia, 115*(1), 102–115. doi:10.1213/ANE.0b013e318253af4b

Segall, N., Hobbs, G., Granger, C. B., Anderson, A. E., Bonifacio, A. S., Taekman, J. M., & Wright, M. C. (2015). Patient load effects on response time to critical arrhythmias in cardiac telemetry: A randomized trial. *Critical Care Medicine, 43*(5), 1036–1042. doi:10.1097/ccm.0000000000000923

Segall, N., Taekman, J. M., Mark, J. B., Hobbs, G. W., & Wright, M. C. (2007). Coding and visualizing eye tracking data in simulated anesthesia care. *Proceedings of the Human Factotrs and Ergonomics Society Annual Meeting, 51*(11), 765–770. doi:10.1177/154193120705101134

Segall, N. S., Wright, M. C., Turner, D. A., Hobbs, G., Maynard, L., & Taekman, J. M. (2011, January 25). *Virtual healthcare environments vs. high-fidelity mannequin-based team training: A comparison of skill acquisition.* Paper presented at the 11th International Meeting on Simulation in Healthcare, New Orleans, LA.

South Australia. Department of Health. Safety and Quality Unit. (2014). *South Australian Patient Safety Report 2012–2013*. Retrieved from http://www.sahealth.sa.gov.au/wps/wcm/connect/7209378046aaedec99a4fb2e504170d4/PSR+12-13+web_PHCS_SQ_20140131.pdf?MOD=AJPERES&CACHEID=7209378046aaedec99a4fb2e504170d4

Steadman, R. H., Berry, A. J., Coursin, D. B., & Andrews, J. J. (2013). Simulation and MOCA®: ASA and ABA perspective: After the first three years. *ASA Newsletter*. Retrieved from http://www.asahq.org/resources/publications/newsletter-articles/2013/august-2013/simulation_and_moca

University of North Carolina at Chapel Hill, Psychology Department. (2008). Counterbalancing in the design of experiments. *Psychology 270 Laboratory Research in Psychology*. Retrieved from http://www.unc.edu/courses/2008spring/psyc/270/001/counterbalancing.html

VA National Center for Patient Safety. (2015). Moderate sedation toolkit for non-anesthesiologists. *VA National Center for Patient Safety Tools*. Retrieved from http://www.patientsafety.va.gov/professionals/onthejob/sedation.asp

Wright, M. C., Breck, S., Evans, J., Ketelhut, K., Lorence, N., Stockman, R., … Landstrom, G. (2014). *Identifying and disseminating best practices in patient monitoring: A human-centered approach*. Paper presented at the 2014 Annual Meeting of the Human Factors and Ergonomics Society, Chicago, IL.

Wright, M. C., Segall, N., Hobbs, G., Phillips-Bute, B., Maynard, L., & Taekman, J. M. (2013). Standardized assessment for evaluation of team skills: Validity and feasibility. *Simulation in Healthcare, 8*(5), 292–303. doi:10.1097/SIH.0b013e318290a022

Wright, M. C., Segall, N., Mark, J. B., Hobbs, G., & Taekman, J. M. (2007). Analyzing and visualizing eye tracking data in simulated anesthesia care. *Anesthesiology, 107*, A1111.

Wright, M. C., & Taekman, J. M. (2003). *Human patient simulators as a human factors research tool in patient safety*. Paper presented at the International Ergonomics Association XVth Triennial Congress and the 7th Joint Conference of the Ergonomics Society of Korea/Japan Ergonomics Society, Seoul Korea.

13

INTERNATIONAL PERSPECTIVES ON THE ROLE OF THE SIMULATION OPERATIONS SPECIALIST

GUILLAUME ALINIER[1] AND ADAM DODSON[2]

[1]*University of Hertfordshire, Hatfield, UK*
[2]*Johns Hopkins Medicine Simulation Center, Baltimore, MD, USA*

The adoption of computer-controlled patient simulators in healthcare education programs can be perceived as having been somewhat slow, despite their relative affordability and successful sales since the beginning of the twenty-first century (Alinier, 2007; Bradley, 2006). One of the often cited obstacles to patient simulator use is their perceived complexity to install, use and troubleshoot, and their acceptance by some learners (pre- or post-qualification or licensure). In addition, some cite the fear of not being able to control the physiological parameters of the simulator in a realistic and timely fashion during a scenario, so the patient simulator behaves like a real human being would. The aforementioned concerns highlight the need for an operator with technical expertise as well as some understanding of clinical practice, human physiology, and pharmacology in order to make the simulator behave appropriately and to, even occasionally, be able to respond to unexpected learner actions (Gantt, 2012). This has rapidly become apparent to many institutions around the world; however, there remains absence of formal career paths and training, despite the growing demand for people with these broad ranging attributes. The importance of preparation and skills mix among the team facilitating a simulation session is emphasized in an article by Lambton and Prion (2009), where it is mentioned that the "faculty" need to

Healthcare Simulation: A Guide for Operations Specialists, First Edition.
Edited by Laura T. Gantt and H. Michael Young.
© 2016 John Wiley & Sons, Inc. Published 2016 by John Wiley & Sons, Inc.

possess educational, clinical, and *technical* expertise. Similar to the real clinical context, where patient care involves the collaboration and contributions of a multi-professional team, the successful facilitation of simulated educational interventions also requires input from professionals with a multitude of skills and attributes. The simulation team may include educational experts, clinicians, psychologists, research scientists, and technologists. This chapter will concentrate on the role of simulation operations specialists (SOS) throughout the world and discuss those who are likely to fulfill simultaneously several of the above mentioned roles. The boundaries are often blurred in terms of roles and responsibilities. It is unlikely that total clarity will be reached by reading this chapter, since the SOS acts as a key resource to the broader simulation team, often fulfilling multiple roles depending on the core simulation team composition and range of simulation-based activities on offer.

THE PLACE FOR SIMULATION OPERATIONS SPECIALISTS AND THEIR CONTRIBUTION TO THE USE OF SIMULATION AROUND THE WORLD

The SOS can be seen as a hybrid professional between the technician and the faculty, often in the position of the simulator operator (Gantt, 2012; Lopreiato & Sawyer, 2015), behind the scenes, but with a key role to play in many aspects of a simulation-based educational encounter with learners. In many institutions, the person occupying this role is seen as the "enabler" in the sense that they have facilitated clinical faculty and learner's access to simulation technology and methodology. Depending on the country, local, or institutional culture, or even seniority, gender, and professional background, the expectations from the SOS's role and contributions to the learners' experience can vary greatly.

Ideally, the role of an SOS should be one of anticipation, responsiveness, ingenuity, innovation, problem-solving, and collaboration for simulation program development. In most places around the globe, operations specialists find themselves fixing things or assisting colleagues finding out "how to ..." quite often. This could be about how to integrate a task trainer made of ballistics gel to supplementing a patient simulator requiring an ultrasound scan in a trauma scenario, or explaining the functionality of a pericardiocentesis task trainer to new faculty. Globally, most SOSs practice on a daily basis the definition of "... and other duties as assigned" often seen in job descriptions. They also need to keep up with technological advances, vendor solutions, equipment maintenance, and various other challenges associated with a nascent function in an evolving domain. It looks like a role shift with the persons who used to or may still be called "Simulation Center Coordinator" or "Simulation Technician" a decade ago, often with an engineering or technical primary qualification, and for whom the scope of practice is now more narrowly defined as either an administrative or technical function.

CHALLENGES FACED BY SIMULATION OPERATIONS SPECIALISTS OR "ANY OTHER DUTIES AND ACTIVITIES AS IDENTIFIED BY THEIR LINE MANAGER"

Internationally, job descriptions are usually quite specific for clinical positions, but when it comes to healthcare simulation professionals, job descriptions are a challenge to write. The cultural or economic context, the power of workers' unions, and local regulations may have a significant impact on the content, details, and expected accuracy of job descriptions. Male and female roles vary at the international level as well. Human resources (HR) departments have specific and different ethical roles and may not always be the best advocates for employees. On the other extreme, HR departments are sometimes perceived as being overprotective and potentially hinder the expected functions of the SOS role, which is something the person in the role can either ignore or play with to their "advantage," or so they might think; it can play against them in terms of team atmosphere, professional development, and creativity.

There are different schools of thought about what skill set is required from an SOS, each with their pros and cons. Most often the argument comes down to whether to hire an employee with a clinical background and then develop their technical abilities, or vice versa. Describing this in a job description may cause significant problems for the HR department for the grading of the position with regard to the expected primary qualification of the potential candidates. It is common for clinical, technical, clerical/administrative, and even academic roles to be linked to different salaries for a similar grade or functions. This implies that, ultimately, the role and duties of the person recruited will be identical, irrespective of whether they have a clinical or technical primary qualification, and yet they may be placed on different salary scales and have different benefits. With regard to the gradual development of a role in relation to the initially expected duties, the person's strengths will generally influence the activities they will engage in and how they will perform. As long as "other duties" are in line with the key objectives of their role, allowing someone to work on tasks in which they excel may be the best approach to adopt in order to get the best from that person.

The challenges of international approaches to HR management and operationalization are the same as they are in the United States. Job descriptions vary greatly for an SOS. HR departments, while mediating between applicants and line managers, can complicate things. The strict adherence to qualifications do not allow for experience or "in lieu of" academic credentials. SOS job candidates may not have a clinical or technical field experience, yet possess skills that could compliment the simulation team. Networking mannequins and pulling data from them or monitoring devices is a challenge commonly faced in some institutions for research purposes. The skills and know-how to complete these tasks are advanced, challenging, and have no specific credentials linked to them, as it is quite specialized.

Along the same line as preparing for the unknown in terms of the actual expected qualities of the candidate recruited, the advertised job itself might be difficult to define; hence the easiest approach is to be very inclusive by making the job description as broad as possible. The roles and responsibilities of the SOS group are ill-defined, as it is still a nascent set of positions varying greatly from institution to institution, and from continent to continent. Through their careers, operations specialists will learn so much that they may become indistinguishable from subject matter experts in domains distant from their initial qualification and credentials. Overall, the SOS is a person from whom much is expected and who significantly contributes to the success of a simulation program in all aspects, including program reputation, financial stability, learning outcomes, development of innovative solutions, and research (Alinier, Pozzo, & Shields, 2008).

Keeping Up with Educational Technologies, Vendor Solutions, and Tools to Maintain Equipment

There are many tools and resources available to maintain knowledge and develop proficiency in relation to the role of an SOS. This can be further enhanced through professional development activities such as attending conferences, workshops, and other courses offered by well-established simulation centers (ASPE, 2015; ASPiH, 2015; INACSL, 2015a; SESAM, 2015; SimGhosts, 2015; SSH, 2015a). Some simulation technology vendors have courses on repair or preventative maintenance of specific simulators. Similarly, companies that offer software-based solutions for the operational aspect of a center or for screen-based simulation also run courses for simulation center staff in administrative and educational positions. Scholarly articles, books, blogs, simulation forums, and websites are also valuable resources to keep up to date with this fast-paced industry (Behind the Sim Curtain, 2015; HealthySim, 2015; KeyIn (formerly Konsiderate) 2015). Social media such as Twitter™ and LinkedIn™ allow vendors and simulation experts from around the world to inform their followers of key developments and events. The Internet and YouTube™, in particular, can be seen as a repository of videos on "how to" and "how not to" resolve a number of issues that the SOS will face. However, not all institutions have the budget to subscribe to online resources or to send staff to courses or international conferences for professional development. Similarly, it is important to note that technology is not always required or even pivotal to facilitating an effective simulation-based training activity, as existing resources often have the potential to be used in a slightly different way to make the learning experience more lifelike or to address different learning objectives (Alinier, 2012; Alinier & Platt, 2014; Tun, Alinier, Tang, & Kneebone, 2015).

Keeping Up with Simulation-Education Practices Institutionally

The SOS is likely to be the common denominator or constant across several simulation program teams within an institution. Implicitly, this places the SOS in a unique position in terms of potential influence and adoption of international simulation education best practices. As a result, the SOS has a form of quality control responsibility, which provides the ability to cross-fertilize good simulation-education and research practices between programs. Valuable guidance can be obtained from key simulation societies in terms of standards of programs, educators, and SOSs (SSH, 2015c), but also with regard to terminology (INACSL, 2015b; SSH, 2015b, 2015c). When the facilities of a simulation center are used by multiple organizations or hospitals, this further extends the reach and impact of the SOS in terms of standardizing good simulation practices, and broadens their experience on a personal level, which, in turn, is beneficial for all simulation programs linked with the SOS's facility.

Keeping Up with Simulation-Education Practices Globally

Although standards exist (SSH, 2015b), they are not always followed and allow for some flexibility; hence, simulation practices vary depending on institution, state, region, county, or country. Some of the variability is due to financial resources, while some could be due to cultural, political, or leadership philosophy about the benefits of simulation or how one exposes oneself to potential critics. Simulations in some countries are called exercises. What is known and what is seen in every corner of the world demonstrate that cultural and fiscal issues impact practice and application of how simulation is utilized. CPR and resuscitation science has been using simulation, task trainers, and mannequins for several decades (Grenvik & Schaefer, 2004). While it may not be referred to as "simulation" within these events, they are still relying on simulation to transfer learning, elevate practice, and demonstrate competency. Other parts of the world are changing practices and pushing the limits of the high acuity intensive care simulation scenarios.

In the world of the SOS, *collaboration* is more important than *competition*. Staying ahead or even keeping up with simulation practices and technology is important, as it contributes to the success of a simulation program in terms of its credibility and quality of the learning that it facilitates. Maintaining currency with the literature is a good way to do this, although there can be significant delays of dissemination of new technology or practices linked with the editing and publishing process of books and the peer review process of journal articles. Social media sites like LinkedIn, SimConnect, Facebook, Twitter, or others give the simulation professional resources to find information, ask questions, and explore answers to a variety of challenging problems and new developments. Alternatively, many websites set up by individuals or groups of like-minded people with an interest in simulation provide useful information and are regularly updated (Behind the Sim Curtain, 2015; Healthy Simulation, 2015; SimGHOSTS, 2015).

An external mark of recognition for one's ability to maintain abreast in a professional field can be demonstrated by the attainment of the certified status as "CHSOS" (Certified Healthcare Simulation Operations Specialist) and even "CHSE" or (CHSE-A) (Certified Healthcare Simulation Educator—Advanced) (SSH, 2015c). The latter credential is particularly relevant to people whose primary function is to facilitate learning through simulation, rather than knowing how to actually set up, run, and trouble shoot the simulator, which would correspond more to the CHSOS certification. These certifications are mutually exclusive and some people could rightfully qualify for both.

Low-Cost Solutions to Enhance Simulation-Based Education without Negatively Affecting Educational Objectives and Outcomes

Often, low-cost solutions can be used to enhance simulation-based education in a more effective way than with the use of more advanced and expensive solutions in the sense that they do not negatively impact on educational outcomes and help achieve the same result from an educational perspective. An SOS usually works with educators, physicians, or nursing staff to complete a needs assessment of the target learner population (see Chapter 7). The needs assessment helps set specific learning objectives around which the scenarios or the practical learning experience is designed (Lioce et al., 2015). In turn, this helps determine the modality that should be used and the level of fidelity required for the simulated experience to be valuable and not overly distracting (Tun et al., 2015). For example, to enhance the simulation of a neurological emergency for a patient in disseminated intravascular coagulation, having the patient's gums and nose bleeding, would be considered important, but no mannequin offers both of these features. It is, however, possible to make some small alterations to create these features on any mannequin with due care for not causing any damage due to fluid spills on electrical components. Similarly, if an identified need is to expose a learner population to an advanced case of Ebola, one would need to think how to make it realistic, since no interactive mannequin can simulate this appropriately at the touch of a button. The most effective solution is probably to resort to moulage by applying make-up on the mannequin (Smith-Stoner, 2011) or a simulated patient (SP). As a word of caution, the moulage should first be tested over a period on a sample of the mannequin's skin to ensure it can still be easily removed even after it has dried. As a useful hint, one should be informed that the local application of a thin layer of wax usually helps prevent any makeup or moulage being absorbed by the skin of the mannequin and potentially creating a permanent stain.

Several low-cost solutions that make a significant difference to the realism of scenarios or act as cues for particular cases are available online through the simulation community and some have been published in books, journal articles, and even websites or blogs (Alinier, 2008a; Merica, 2011; Smith-Stoner, 2011; Swan, 2013). Some of these solutions are presented below.

SIMULATION INNOVATIONS

Many individuals who qualify for the title of SOS have greatly contributed to a number of innovations (Alfa-Wali & Antoniou, 2011; Alinier, 2008b, 2008c; Barrier, Thompson, McCullough, & Occhino, 2012; Hong et al., 2012; Lighthall & Harrison, 2010; Taylor, 2008). The results of their efforts are often not visible to the wider simulation community and remain confined to their institution. Opportunities for innovators to share their work exist during international conferences, such as the International Meeting for Simulation in Healthcare IMSH, where awards are allocated to the best innovations (Various Authors, 2012). Below is a series of such innovations is various aspects of simulation.

Possible Enhancements to Simulators and Standardized Patients

Patient Monitoring   In low resource settings, or to overcome technical constraints, several solutions can be used to allow patient monitoring with a mannequin or standardized patient even if one does not have an actual patient monitor and the required sensors and attachments that link the patient to the monitor. The principle is to emulate the patient monitor and the information it provides care givers, and to allow convey key information to run the scenario in a realistic manner.

The first solution is creating a series of screen captures with the desired physiological parameters for the scenario and printing them out. As the scenario evolves, the printouts are displayed to the learners in place of the patient monitor. The second solution allows for more improvisation and "on the fly" changes to the physiological parameters of the patient. It requires on operator and relies on using a computer monitor in lieu of the patient monitor. Depending on the local programming expertise and resources available, this can be done with a normal personal computer with Microsoft PowerPoint™, for example, or a laptop with an additional monitor used to display the extended desktop in "presentation mode." In the latter configuration described, as the scenario progresses, the monitor that faces the learners can be updated with the appropriate monitoring information (Zegezottel, 2013). Animated graphics or still images can be incorporated for the electrocardiograph, colored text boxes can be used to present vital signs, and upon the request of scenario participants the operator will be able to provide X-ray images and blood gases, for example (Alinier, 2008c). A third solution is to use the emulated monitoring capability of a computer-controlled patient simulator without actually using the corresponding mannequin. This sometimes corresponds to using the software as connecting to a "virtual" simulator. The fourth solution is to use an application, some of which are free, that helps connect two tablets, one acting as the instructor control tablet to select the physiological parameters (input device), and the other one representing the patient monitor (output device) with the selected vital signs (DART Sim, 2014) (Fig. 13.1).

Often the learning objectives are not focused on the vital sign changes but on the assessment, so the very accurate and continuous update of vital signs with a running rhythm is not necessarily crucial. The old saying "treat the patient, not the monitor" can often be enforced due to financial constraints or simply as it is not a crucial aspect of realism that requires total fidelity (Tun et al., 2015). The question that one should ask when preparing the simulation environment is "Is the full functionality of the patient monitor a necessity in relation to any of the learning objectives set for this scenario?"

Central Venous Pressure Monitoring   Another aspect of patient monitoring that requires a particular calibration process when performed in a traditional manner and that can be taught using simulation is central venous pressure (CVP) monitoring. The result of this invasive process is usually simply represented as a value on an emulated patient simulator monitor. This, however, limits the learning opportunities with fundamental aspects of CVP calibration and monitoring. A relatively simple setup

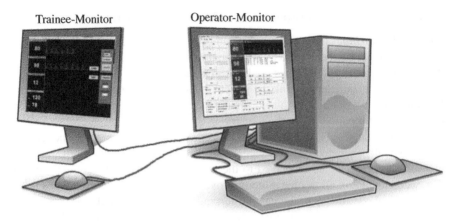

FIGURE 13.1 Representation of the Vital Sign Simulator configuration on a personal computer with two graphics card outputs (Zegezottel, 2013).

has been described in a book chapter by Alinier (2008b) and could prove a valuable way of teaching important critical care aspects of CVP monitoring.

Moulage   SOSs are often the experts in moulage or make up to simulate wounds, injuries, or other physical signs linked to disease or skin lesions. Whether it be a femur fracture, cervical spine step-off, or simply simulating phlebitis, moulage can be very important to the level of fidelity of a scenario to generate a reaction from scenario participants. Moulage of internal organs or external wounds can be developed for a scenario of a trauma patient going to surgery, and involving a multidisciplinary team (e.g. physicians, nurses, technicians, clergy, security, radiology). Not only is moulage important as a visual cue, but it can be just as important to the other senses as well. One may add Gatorade to simulated urine for positive result to sugar testing in maternity scenarios. Odors can also be used to simulate the smell of gangrene. Effort in moulage is usually correlated to the learning objectives; hence, if none of the objectives are directly affected by the realism of the injury, the moulage can remain basic.

Ballistic Gel Usage Throughout Multiple Disciplines   Ballistic gel or even gelatin has been used in many countries to create molded task trainers for under US$50.00 that can be used for ultrasound scanning. The benefits of this low cost, high usage capability are essential in many countries. The molds made can be used in multiple disciplines and reused. The cost of this approach is as low as US$1.00 to US$3.00 per item as opposed to a product on the market which can cost several thousand US dollars.

Standardized and Simulated Patients   The use of standardized and simulated patients (SPs) in healthcare education has been very common practice for several decades (Barrows, 1993; Boulet et al., 1998; Levine & Swartz, 2008; Norman,

Tugwell, & Feightner, 1982; Stillman, Swanson, & Smee, 1986). SPs can be perceived as a low-resource country solution to offering scenario-based learning, as it is an approach that can help avoid the purchase of training equipment. SP use can even be sometimes wrongly perceived as a subdomain or lesser form of simulation than simulation using so-called high-fidelity patient simulators. However, both clearly have a place in the educational continuum and, in many respects, the use of a live person is more realistic than a mannequin of any degree of fidelity (Alinier, 2007; Chiniara et al., 2013; Collins & Harden, 1998; Tun et al., 2015). Despite not necessarily involving the use of technology, the SOS can play a critical role in the effective use of SPs. The SOS often has the ability to take the role of an SP or to brief someone as to how they should act to portray the chosen case because they have the educational understanding underpinning the experience to which learners need to be exposed to demonstrate predetermined learning outcomes. Another aspect to which the SOS may bring a particular understanding is when standardized or simulated patients need to be supplemented by technology to help simulate particular signs or symptoms, or to allow for the practice of invasive clinical skills (Nestel, Kneebone, & Black, 2006). This may, for example, involve the use of a stethoscope simulator with which the SP has to press a button depending on where the clinician is placing the stethoscope in order to play a prerecorded sound potentially synchronized with the patient's heart or breathing rate (Verma, Bhatt, Booton, & Kneebone, 2011).

Possible Enhancements to the Simulation Environment

In situ Learning in Austere Environments   Several facilities, schools, and institutions use *in situ* settings as the training environment. "In situ" is a Latin term for "in the natural or original place;" in the context of healthcare simulation-based education, this can be any real clinical environment corresponding to the case, or even a pre-hospital care setting inside a house or on the street for community nurses, family physicians, or paramedics (Hssain, Alinier, & Souaiby, 2013; Patterson, Blike, & Nadkarni, 2008).

An austere environment can be defined as an area that regularly experiences environmental or human hazards, such as extreme weather or regular acts of violence, or an area with limited access to basic resources or utilities such as electricity and drinking water. Conducting simulation in such environments often goes beyond some of the expectations that simulation should be conducted in a "safe and controlled" environment. Aspects of austere environments can be "uncontrollable" as opposed to simulations in more traditional settings. The lessons derived from such experiences can be very powerful, but are not without dangers and do not necessarily allow for all expected learning objectives to be achieved.

Many austere environments present limitations such as regular power outages, equipment thefts, and security or safety risks. In doing *in situ* simulation in such environments, measures need to be taken to try and control some of the environmental factors which may only be achievable, thanks to the use of additional manpower and equipment. Another factor that goes against recommended simulation design standards (Lioce et al., 2015) is that these environments require more flexibility and the willingness to improvise while still ensuring unique and valuable learning can be derived from it. This is where the versatility and adaptability skills of an SOS in overcoming difficulties can greatly contribute to the success of a simulation.

Language Barriers   In some settings, such as *in situ* simulation or simulation in austere environments, learning objectives related to communication issues linked to language differences are relatively common. Such aspects of human factors can be linked to culture, geography, nationality, or ethnicity and can be an important and highly relevant factor in which to expose learners. Working through a translator either in the form of another learner, or as a confederate or actor, is something to be experienced. Some speak simultaneously (and keep up!). Others function by having what is to be translated spoken and then translate.

Another aspect to consider is when an SOS is involved in international work. Whether the environment is considered austere or not, language differences will always affect the pace of work, so good time management is a must. Communication difficulties can be expected to double the normal duration of a regular session. If interpreters are required but unavailable, resorting to pictorial aids or repeated demos can be very beneficial. Even if half a day is spent with the interpreter to go through the program of activities and contents of any teaching material, it will help that person better understand the core concepts and messages to be passed on. Ultimately, it will help that person provide a better service during the actual training day(s) and help save time.

Improving Simulation Center Operations   The SOS with the right skills will directly benefit the operations of a simulation center in various areas. For example, the background running of a simulation center by developing a website that allows for sessions, rooms, and equipment bookings is one way the SOS may do this. Another example that has revolutionized the way some institutions run their Objective Structured Clinical Examination (OSCE) was the development of an automated computer-based OSCE clock system, allowing for the simultaneous display of the timer and voice prompts on multiple networked monitors in an OSCE facility (Alinier & Dodd, 2007). This kind of setup helps minimize the manpower required to run an OSCE in an organized manner. Figure 13.2 illustrates how the OSCE timer used at the University of Hertfordshire is programmed and operates.

RESEARCH BY SIMULATION OPERATIONS SPECIALISTS AROUND THE GLOBE

Many SOSs are undoubtedly involved in conducting or even leading research projects in their institutions. However, this leadership is difficult to identify since the SOS job title is still relatively new and only appears on a couple of journal articles when performing a Google Scholar search (Lopreiato & Sawyer, 2015; Ottaviano & Washington, 2009). Once the CHSOS certification launched in 2015 by the Society for Simulation in Healthcare (SSH, 2015c) has become more mainstream and that the

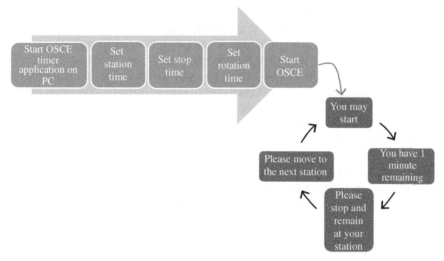

FIGURE 13.2   Representation of the customized OSCE application process.

acronym of this credential is more commonly used, it will be easier to identify when operations specialists are involved as publication authors. Chapter 12 of this book discusses research efforts by a number of operations specialists.

The types of research that the SOS may be involved in can be very broad and encompass such topics as testing of patient safety initiatives, educational research studies, technological developments, and environmental testing. Due to their potentially diverse backgrounds, operations specialists can bring relatively unique skills and different perspective to a research team's efforts. As highlighted earlier in this chapter, the broad knowledge base, creativity, ability to solve problems, and innovative nature makes the SOS a valuable asset on a research team.

From a global perspective, the adoption of the SOS appellation or recognition of the functions of the role may take a long time to spread around the world. Many countries are still at the phase of considering the value of employing "simulation technicians." Some who already have kept them from gaining their due recognition or the opportunity to fully expand in the role by demonstrating their ability to take initiative. This may be due to peer pressure from other "technicians" who wish to stop those who try to differentiate themselves from others or an organizational culture that creates a divide between faculty and support staff. The likely outcome is that it may be sometime before anyone working in an SOS capacity in such settings emerges visibly on the research scene.

CONCLUSION

The nature of the role of the SOS is such that it requires persons who can excel in several domains encompassing education, technology, and clinical practice. From an international perspective, the role is not quite clearly defined and people may perform similar duties under different job titles. Ultimately, however, the role is pivotal in its ability to role that bring safeguards to a simulation program and peace of mind to simulation facilitators and educators (CHSE and CHSE-A). Although there is an increasing focus on the importance of the educational aspects of simulation as a teaching approach, rather than the technology employed, this does not make the role of the SOS redundant. The SOS plays a crucial role as part of a simulation team in many aspects, thanks to the broad range of skills and attributes contributed to various forms of simulation modalities. Whether a simulation program focuses on the use of standardized patients, virtual reality surgical simulators, or full-body patient simulators, the SOS always has a role to play. Globally, despite potential local "oppression," the person in such a role needs to be given due recognition and autonomy to express their abilities in order to be used to their full potential, which may also include teaching, whether through briefing and/or debriefing, and research activities.

REFERENCES

Alfa-Wali, M., & Antoniou, A. (2011). Eco-friendly laparoscopic home trainer. *Simulation in Healthcare, 6*(3), 176–179. doi:10.1097/SIH.0b013e318208549b

Alinier, G. (2007). A typology of educationally focused medical simulation tools. *Medical Teacher, 29*(8), e243–250.

Alinier, G. (2008a). How to create clinical environments out of smoke and mirrors. In R. R. Kyle & W. B. Murray (Eds.), *Clinical simulation: Operations, engineering, and management* (1st ed., pp. 701–712). San Diego, CA: Academic Press.

Alinier, G. (2008b). Professional stage craft: How to create simulated clinical environments out of smoke and mirrors. In R. R. Kyle & W. B. Murray (Eds.), *Clinical simulation: Operations, engineering, and management* (1st ed., pp. 515–516). San Diego, CA: Academic Press.

Alinier, G. (2008c). *A touch of added realism: Simulated electronic patient record monitor.* Paper presented at the 14th Conference of the Society in Europe for Simulation Applied to Medicine, Hatfield, UK.

Alinier, G. (2012). Push for the provision of technology enhanced learning... with what you can afford! *International Paramedic Practice, 1*(2), 153–154.

Alinier, G., & Dodd, P. (2007). *Computerised multi-location OSCE timing system.* Paper presented at the Annual Meeting of the National Association of Medical Simulators, 6–7 September 2007, Hatfield, UK.

Alinier, G., & Platt, A. (2014). International overview of high-level simulation education initiatives in relation to critical care. *Nursing in Critical Care, 19*(1), 42–49. doi:10.1111/nicc.12030

Alinier, G., Pozzo, R., & Shields, C. (2008). The simulation professional: Gets things done and attracts opportunities. In R. R. Kyle & W. B. Murray (Eds.), *Clinical simulation: Operations, engineering, and management* (1st ed., pp. 507–511). San Diego, CA: Academic Press.

ASPE. (2015). *Association of Standardized Patient Educators.* Retrieved April 16, 2015 from http://www.aspeducators.org

ASPiH. (2015). *Association for Simulated Practice in Healthcare.* Retrieved April 16, 2015 from http://www.aspih.org.uk/

Barrier, B. F., Thompson, A. B., McCullough, M. W., & Occhino, J. A. (2012). A novel and inexpensive vaginal hysterectomy simulator. *Simulation in Healthcare, 7*(6), 374–379. doi:10.1097/SIH.0b013e318266d0c6

Barrows, H. S. (1993). An overview of the uses of standardized patients for teaching and evaluating clinical skills. AAMC. *Academic Medicine, 68*(6), 443–451; discussion 451–443.

Behind the Sim Curtain. (2015). *Do you work "Behind the Sim Curtain"?* Retrieved April 16, 2015 from http://www.behindthesimcurtain.com/

Boulet, J. R., Ben-David, M. F., Ziv, A., Burdick, W. P., Curtis, M., Peitzman, S., & Gary, N. E. (1998). Using standardized patients to assess the interpersonal skills of physicians. *Academic Medicine, 73*(10 Suppl), S94–96.

Bradley, P. (2006). The history of simulation in medical education and possible future directions. *Medical Education, 40*(3), 254–262.

Chiniara, G., Cole, G., Brisbin, K., Huffman, D., Cragg, B., Lamacchia, M., … Canadian Network For Simulation In Healthcare, Guidelines Working Group. (2013). Simulation in healthcare: A taxonomy and a conceptual framework for instructional design and media selection. *Medical Teacher, 35*(8), e1380–1395. doi:10.3109/0142159X.2012.733451

Collins, J. P., & Harden, R. M. (1998). AMEE medical education guide no. 13: Real patients, simulated patients and simulators in clinical examinations. *Medical Teacher, 20*(6), 508–521.

DART Sim. (2014). *DART ECG Simulator.* Retrieved April 24, 2015 from http://ecg-simulator.com/

Gantt, L. (2012). Who's driving? The role and training of the human patient simulation operator. *Computers, Informatics, Nursing, 30*(11), 579–586.

Grenvik, A., & Schaefer, J. (2004). From Resusci-Anne to Sim-Man: The evolution of simulators in medicine. *Critical Care Medicine, 32*(2 Suppl), S56–57.

HealthySim. (2015). *Healthy simulation: Sharing and growing the field of healthcare simulation.* Retrieved April 16, 2015 from http://healthysimulation.com/

Hong, A., Mullin, P. M., Al-Marayati, L., Peyre, S. E., Muderspach, L., Macdonald, H., … Lee, R. H. (2012). A low-fidelity total abdominal hysterectomy teaching model for obstetrics and gynecology residents. *Simulation in Healthcare, 7*(2), 123–126. doi:10.1097/SIH.0b013e31823471bb

Hssain, I., Alinier, G., & Souaiby, N. (2013). In-situ simulation: A different approach to patient safety through immersive training. *Mediterranean Journal of Emergency Medicine, 15*, 17–28.

INACSL. (2015a). *International Nursing Association for Clinical Simulation & Learning.* Retrieved April 16, 2015 from http://www.inacsl.org

INACSL. (2015b). *Standards of best practice: Simulation.* Retrieved May 16, 2015 from http://www.inacsl.org/i4a/pages/index.cfm?pageid=3407

Konsiderate. (2015). *Medical simulation purchase reviews.* Retrieved April 16, 2015 from https://www.konsiderate.com/

Lambton, J., & Prion, S. (2009). The value of simulation in the development of observational skills for clinical microsystems. *Clinical Simulation in Nursing, 5*(4), e137–143.

Levine, A. I., & Swartz, M. H. (2008). Standardized patients: The "other" simulation. *Journal of Critical Care, 23*(2), 179–184. doi:10.1016/j.jcrc.2007.12.001

Lighthall, G. K., & Harrison, T. K. (2010). A controllable patient monitor for classroom video projectors. *Simulation in Healthcare, 5*(1), 58–60. doi:10.1097/SIH.0b013e3181b5c3e6

Lioce, L., Meakim, C., Fey, M. K., Chmil, J. V., Mariani, B., & Alinier, G. (2015). Standards of best practice: Simulation design. *Clinical Simulation in Nursing, 11*, 309–315.

Lopreiato, J. O., & Sawyer, T. (2015). Simulation-based medical education in pediatrics. *Academic Pediatrics, 15*(2), 134–142.

Merica, B. J. (2011). *Medical moulage: How to make your simulations come alive.* Philadelphia, PA: F.A. Davis.

Nestel, D., Kneebone, R., & Black, S. (2006). Simulated patients and the development of procedural and operative skills. *Medical Teacher, 28*, 390–391.

Norman, G. R., Tugwell, P., & Feightner, J. W. (1982). A comparison of resident performance on real and simulated patients. *Journal of Medical Education, 57*(9), 708–715.

Ottaviano, G., & Washington, C. (2009). Northwest simulation center—sharpens clinical and communication skills for individuals and teams. *The Permanente Journal, 13*(2), 37–43.

Patterson, M. D., Blike, G. T., & Nadkarni, V. M. (2008). In situ simulation: Challenges and results. In K. Henriksen, J. B. Battles, M. A. Keyes, & M. L. Grady (Eds.), *New directions and alternative approaches* (Vol. 3. Performance and Tools. AHRQ Publication No. 08-0034-3) (pp. 1–18). Rockville, MD: Agency for Healthcare Research and Quality.

SESAM. (2015). *Society in Europe for Simulation Applied to Medicine.* Retrieved April 16, 2015 from http://www.sesam-web.org

SimGHOSTS. (2015). *SimGHOSTS: Simulation Technology Specialists.* Retrieved April 16, 2015 from http://www.simghosts.org/

Smith-Stoner, M. (2011). Using moulage to enhance educational instruction. *Nurse Educator, 36*(1), 21–24.

SSH. (2015a). *Society for Simulation in Healthcare.* Retrieved April 16, 2015 from http://www.ssih.org/

SSH. (2015b). *SSH Accreditation of Healthcare Simulation Programs.* Retrieved April 16, 2015 from http://www.ssih.org/Accreditation

SSH. (2015c). *SSH Certification Programs.* Retrieved April 16, 2015 from http://www.ssih.org/Certification

Stillman, P. L., Swanson, D. B., & Smee, S. (1986). Assessing clinical skills of residents with standardized patients. *Annals of Internal Medicine, 105*(5), 762–771.

Swan, N. A. (2013). Burn moulage made easy (and cheap). *Journal of Burn Care & Research, 34*(4), e215–220.

Taylor, T. (2008). How to create a clinical data station for use in a high fidelity medical simulation lab. *Simulation in Healthcare, 3*(2), 128–130. doi:10.1097/SIH.0b013e31815a8af4

Tun, J. K., Alinier, G., Tang, J., & Kneebone, R. L. (2015). Redefining Simulation Fidelity for Healthcare Education. *Simulation & Gaming, (In press)*, 1–16.

Various Authors. (2012). Technology Innovations to be Presented at the 13th Annual International Meeting on Simulation in Healthcare: January 26th–30th, 2013 Orlando, Florida. *Simulation in Healthcare, 7*(6), 546–569. doi:10.1097/SIH.0b013e31827e77e6

Verma, A., Bhatt, H., Booton, P., & Kneebone, R. (2011). The Ventriloscope(R) as an innovative tool for assessing clinical examination skills: Appraisal of a novel method of simulating auscultatory findings. *Medical Teacher, 33*(7), e388–396. doi:10.3109/0142159X.2011.579200

Zegezottel. (2013). *Vital Sign Simulator.* Retrieved April 24, 2015 from http://sourceforge.net/projects/vitalsignsim/

14

PROFESSIONAL DEVELOPMENT FOR THE NEXT GENERATION OF SIMULATION OPERATIONS SPECIALISTS

THOMAS A. DONGILLI

Winter Institute for Simulation Education and Research (WISER), Pittsburgh, PA, USA

INTRODUCTION

As education and healthcare change, so do the roles of the simulation operations specialists (SOS). Some programs consist of one person doing everything; other programs consist of a team with detailed roles and responsibilities. Whatever the location and role, the SOS will need to anticipate growth and change. Staying current with these changes can be a challenge. The SOS must stay involved in continuing education in the industry, interacting with the healthcare simulation community, and staying apprised of new technology and best practices. This chapter discusses the various roles of the SOS and how to plan for an ever-changing future.

TRADITIONAL MODELS OF OPERATION

In recent history, traditional models of operation for the SOS consisted of an instructor teaching with the SOS providing support. That support would consist of room preparation, scenario programming, and support during the actual class. However, many operations specialists became involved in the academic, operations, administrative

Healthcare Simulation: A Guide for Operations Specialists, First Edition.
Edited by Laura T. Gantt and H. Michael Young.
© 2016 John Wiley & Sons, Inc. Published 2016 by John Wiley & Sons, Inc.

and research sides of simulation programs as well, though many operations specialists had no experience in these areas or possessed limited skills in a few of them. Hence, the primary focus of the SOS was on support of the center and its courses. This led to very vague job descriptions within the industry because job functionality was based on the specific location and role requirements within a center. As a result, seeking assistance, education, and training was difficult for the SOS as responsibilities varied from center to center. Early education was based on what was learned from vendor led inservices, training, and conferences.

As programs grew in numbers, so did the role of the SOS. Responsibilities like scheduling and calendar management, process oversight, inventory control, development of policies and procedures, and other administrative functions all became part of the standard requirements for the position. The need for role standardization was accelerated each year. Some centers created programs to train their own operations specialists. These programs were typically biased toward that center's operational model. Even though these efforts benefited the SOS community, an industry standard was still missing.

In 2014 Society for Simulation in Healthcare (SSH) introduced the Certified Healthcare Simulation Operations Specialists (CHSOS). The CHSOS program was designed to create an industry standard for centers and SOS professionals. An SOS seeking the CHSOS should prepare for an examination that, if passed, demonstrates minimal competencies for the SOS workforce and endeavors to provide the first real standardization of the various roles of the SOS profession. This certification will be discussed in more detail later in the chapter.

THE EXPANDING ROLE OF THE SOS

The role of the SOS has expanded exponentially over the past 3 years. Factors that contribute to this expansion include loss of faculty time to teach, budget constraints, and an increased awareness of a need to supply simulation data and proof of value, forcing the SOS to integrate more within programs. Many programs now utilize the SOS in a more integrated role.

There was a time when the role of the SOS was limited to the technical operations of a center. Now, many find themselves involved in all aspects of simulation including curriculum development, administration, teaching, debriefing, assessment, and research. With these expanding roles of the SOS, there has been an associated escalation of responsibilities. Many of these responsibilities contribute to the overall management and operations of a center. It makes sense that responsibilities like scheduling and process management, equipment purchases, and operations and associated administrative duties be incorporated into the role of the SOS. Many programs have now created a coordinator, managerial or operations director role for the person overseeing these responsibilities.

Many operations specialists have been integral in the development of curriculum and education, including assisting course authors in scenario design, matching the appropriate equipment with the learning objectives, and training facilitators on how to use the equipment, hardware and software. Educating new instructors how to operate and utilize the simulator hardware and software, or assisting with the development of scenarios, are all considered forms of teaching. Program policies and regulatory agencies define who is allowed to teach students; this is an area of needed awareness for the SOS. Some programs have created formal "Course Director or Course Instructor" training programs, designed to educate personnel new to these roles. The SOS plays a key role in the development and teaching of these programs. An easy way to start such a program is to the have the SOS document processes for training of instructors or course directors, then have them create a formal curriculum pertaining to this. The benefit of such a project would be to allow the SOS to understand the process of curriculum development while creating a formal program for director and instructor training. Even if the SOS is not directly involved in the curriculum development process, they should be made aware of it and be included when it comes time to select resources such as simulators, rooms, medical equipment, supplies, and scenario programming.

Even though simulation centers are diverse in their missions and populations that they serve, most still have some common or core programs that are offered by many. Obtaining certification in BLS, ACLS, or PALS could benefit the SOS for many reasons. For the SOS who comes from a more technical background, one or more of these certification courses allow the SOS to learn some clinical concepts, terminology, and basic physiology. For those SOSs who have a health-care background, it is another certification or standard that can be utilized to assure the SOS team is maintaining clinical knowledge and aware of current guidelines and best practices.

Another area that most overlook, but are actively involved in, is research. The SOS plays a key role in almost all research projects that occur in a simulation center. Data management is critical to a research study. The SOS should assist with identification of the tools needed to collect and organize the data, standardizing room configurations, training of evaluators on simulation center equipment being utilized for the study, and how data will be stored or accessed once a study or session has been completed. The involvement of the SOS should happen early in the design of a study that utilizes a simulation center, even before institutional review board (IRB) approval is sought. This will allow the primary investigator (PI) of a research study and the simulation center to match the appropriate equipment and software to the study. Once the equipment and software have been identified, the involvement level of the SOS should be determined. Typical SOS involvement includes the following: (i) an initial meeting with the PI to review the simulation center resources, which should include the center's AV, IT, simulators task trainers, facilities (rooms), and medical equipment available; (ii) a review of the support levels of the SOS in the development of the project, which topics should include instructor training and scenario programming; (iii) in the planning phase of the event, review the expectations and level of SOS support for that day, which should include equipment preparation, data collection, data storage, and form completion (paperwork); (iv) the last part of the planning process should address how data will be collected, analyzed, reported, and migrated out of the center.

CERTIFICATION

In 2014, the SSH launched the Certified Healthcare Simulation Operations Specialist or CHSOS professional certification program (http://www.ssih.org/ Certification/CHSOS). The intent of the program is to formalize the role of the SOS as well as establish a clear measurement of competencies required to perform in such a position. Professional development including certifications like the CHSOS will play a fundamental role in the future of the SOS community. Programs created to support CHSOS or affiliated programs should be governed by similar or same continuing education credits CME/CE requirements that the industry is accustomed to. The development of continuing educational programs for CHSOS preparation will contribute to the design of formalized educational programs, thus advancing simulation in general. Grants and funding would be more likely to go to programs where staff members have such certifications. In addition, the standard is now set for what simulation professionals believe are the minimal requirements for functioning as an SOS. It may be time for each operations specialist to consider what all of this means.

The SOS role is dynamic; 1 minute there is a technical issue to troubleshoot, while the next is spent designing a scenario with an instructor. With the diversity of knowledge and skills required of the role, and the reality that some operations specialists come from a more technical, less healthcare-related background, the SOS group now needs to be technical and medical because of the recognized need for integration of the SOS into more aspects of center operations and course development. As was discussed earlier, one initial solution to this issue could be to obtain BLS certification. Once some experience with this certification is achieved, BLS instructor certification could be pursued as well. This will help with two primary functions: it allows the non-medical person to get some understanding of medicine and becoming an instructor helps with understanding what it takes to teach a course and debrief an individual or team. Such certifications could also allow the SOS to further their role in the curriculum development process. Those who have existing ACLS certification, becoming an ACLS instructor, will have an added benefit.

For those operations specialists that hold professional licenses, such as EMT, RT or RN or those involved in the teaching and curriculum development process, the SSH has also created professional certification programs for advancing the field of healthcare educators with the Certified Healthcare Simulation Educator (CHSE) and the CHSE-A (advanced) programs (http://www.ssih.org/Certification/CHSE).

Both of these certifications are geared toward those individuals interested in obtaining certification as a simulation educator. For those operations specialists who have multiple roles as educator, SOS, and curriculum developer, this certification may be beneficial. Even if an SOS does not function in all of these roles, the certification will help the SOS to have a better understanding of the processes and work that is required to create and teach courses.

CONTINUING EDUCATION EFFORTS

As an SOS, there are many ways to continue one's education. Attend training sessions that count toward certification or relate directly toward expanding job functionality. With increasing involvement in this growing profession, training and educational opportunities will be easier to find since many simulation centers offer programs. With budgets being closely monitored, the SOS must consider programs that may contribute toward licensure or certification. If neither of these are a concern, select programs that would allow advancement of skills as an SOS or introduce new concepts for personal or professional development. Many simulation centers offer programs pertaining to curriculum development, instructor training, scenario programming, debriefing, and so on. Choose opportunities from comparable simulation programs to best meet specific training needs. Talk to people who have taken specific courses and get feedback.

Another way to meet continuing education needs could be through regional, national, and international simulation meetings, such as the International Meeting for Simulation in Healthcare (IMSH), the International Nursing Association for Clinical Simulation and Learning (INACSL), or any of the dozens of SSH affiliates. Most of these meetings have an annual meeting some with a few hundred attendees, and some, like IMSH, where thousands of attendees come to network and participate in workshops, lectures, meetings, and demonstrations, all pertaining to the field of healthcare simulation. The conference content is usually divided by topics that are of most interest to the members. Some of the topics include curriculum design, research, team training, administration and, more recently, operations.

For those who have issues with travel budgets or time constraints, webinars can provide a cost effective way to obtain continuing education credits. Some simulation centers and even the SSIH offer such programs http://www.ssih.org/Accreditation/Webinar-Library. These programs usually last an hour or less and can be attended by simply logging in and participating.

Regional and local meetings are another way to get continuing education. Stay in communication with regional and local simulation centers and vendors. Most will know of conferences or workshops that may be within driving distance. Vendor-led workshops are a great way to learn how to utilize their products and see new products; however, these events are typically for the novice user of their products, and do not go much further into the SOSs professional training needs. There are, however, some vendors that offer more in-depth training programs. Such programs are generally taught by current users of the products and demonstrate how the product was integrated or utilized at a particular center. This is a great way to see and hear the work of others who may use similar products.

No matter what the event, whether a workshop or conference, plan on networking and increasing a personal database of resources. Make an effort to locate local, state, regional, and national resources.

PROFESSIONAL ADVANCEMENT

How does the SOS manage processes at a center? How does the SOS train instructors or program scenarios? These are all things the SOS probably does on a regular basis, but may never have shared with anyone. Publications and presentations can be a great way to share work with others. Publications come in the form of abstracts, news stories, articles, books, and book chapters. Presentations can be done locally (to internal or external groups), regionally, nationally, and internationally. Before considering any presentation or publication, the SOS should begin by documenting simulation center processes. Forms may be used to help with documentation and these forms may be cited within the publication as well. The SOS must be prepared to defend or explain processes and why they were created, what problem or inefficiency they solved. Once work processes are documented, the next step is identification of the appropriate venue to present or submit. Some journals will not accept technically oriented submissions, while others will. Research is required to determine what venue best matches a submission or presentation. These may include the *Simulation in Healthcare* and Medsim magazine (halldale.com/medsim).

In addition to publications and presentations, professional societies provide opportunities for getting involved and networking also. Being new to a group, the SOS may begin as a presenter or guest lecturer. As experience grows within a society, so do advancement opportunities. An active member has a chance to make a difference. Getting involved will allow expansion of professional networks, as well as academic and professional experiences.

CONCLUSION

As healthcare simulation changes and grows, so will the role of the SOS. SOSs must look for ways to expand their current roles, as well as anticipate the future. The SOS should take a moment to assess their various programs and see where each program is heading in the next few years. Does the operations specialists' skill set match the vision and the preparation required? If not, what will it take to get there? Striving toward the competencies identified in certifications like the CHSOS or CHSE can be a great way to not only obtain basic knowledge, but also stay in communication with healthcare simulation standards and best practices through continuing education and maintenance of such certifications. Stay involved by presenting at or attending conferences as well; these provide additional venues to learn, network, and define the career paths of current and future SOSs.

APPENDIX 1

COMMONLY USED SIMULATION TERMS, TERMINOLOGY, AND MEDICAL ABBREVIATIONS

LAURA T. GANTT[1] AND H. MICHAEL YOUNG[2]

[1]*East Carolina University College of Nursing, Greenville, NC, USA*
[2]*Level 3 Healthcare, Mesa, AZ, USA*

ABC: Airway, breathing, circulation.

AC: Ante cibum—before a meal.

Advocacy and inquiry: A communication method within debriefing that pairs a statement of observation and point of view (advocacy) with a question directed at understanding an action through a participant's cognitive construct or frame (inquiry) (Palaganas, Maxworthy, Epps, & Mancini, 2015).

AMA: Against medical advice.

APAP: Automatic positive airway pressure; paracetamol (acetaminophen).

Assessment: The process of documenting, usually in measurable terms, a subject's knowledge, skills, attitudes, and beliefs (Levine, DeMaria, & Schwartz, 2013).

Avatar: Graphical representation of the user or user's alter ego or character. It may take either a three-dimensional form, as in games or virtual worlds, or a two-dimensional form as an icon in Internet forums and other online communities.

Behavioral skills: The decision-making and team interaction processes used during team's management of a situation (Gaba et al., 1998).

Best practice: An idea that asserts that there is a technique, method, process, activity, incentive, or reward that is more effective at delivering particular outcomes than any

Healthcare Simulation: A Guide for Operations Specialists, First Edition.
Edited by Laura T. Gantt and H. Michael Young.

other technique, method, process, and so on. Best practices can also be defined as the most efficient (least amount of effort) and effective (best results) way of accomplishing a task based on repeatable procedures that have proven themselves over time for large numbers of people (SSH).

Briefing: This refers to any activity that occurs prior to a simulation event such as an educational activity. This can include giving instructions, guidelines, or directives. Briefings can be for the benefit of the instructional staff as well as for the learner(s) (SSH).

CABG: Coronary artery bypass grafting.

CHF: Congestive heart failure.

CHSE: Certification Healthcare Simulation Educator (SSH).

CHSE-A: Certification Healthcare Simulation Educator-Advanced (SSH).

CHSOS: Certified Healthcare Simulation Operations Specialist (SSH).

CHSOS program: A term used throughout various documents and resources of the CHSOS certification. It is a general term used to encompass any and all activities related to the application, verification, certification granting, administrative, and other functions performed in the certification program (SSH, 2015).

COPD: Chronic obstructive pulmonary disease.

Clinical scenario (also referred to as a simulation scenario, simulated case): A plan of an expected and potential course of events for a simulated clinical experience. The clinical scenario provides the context for the simulation and can vary in length and complexity, depending on the objective. A clinical scenario may include the following components:

- Participant preparation
- Prebriefing (or Briefing): objectives, questions, and/or materials
- Patient information describing the situation to be managed
- Learning objectives
- Environmental conditions, including manikin, patient, embedded simulated person preparation
- Related equipment, props, and tools, and/or resources for assessing and managing the simulated experience, for example, pathology reports, defibrillator
- Expectations, limitations and potential roles of participant
- A progression outline including a beginning and ending
- Debriefing process
- Evaluation criteria (Palaganas et al., 2015).

Computer-based simulation: Simulation activities that are performed via a computer program. These are similar to virtual reality simulations, but do not include additional interfaces between the learner and the computer (restricted to mouse-type interface for example) (SSH).

Confederate: An individual other than the patient who is scripted in a simulation to provide realism, additional challenges, or additional information for the learner (Levine et al., 2013).

Construct validity: Refers to "the degree to which a test measures what it claims, or purports, to be measuring." In other words, it occurs whenever a test is to be interpreted as a measure of some attribute or quality which is not operationally defined. In lay terms, construct validity examines the question: "does the measure behave like the theory says a measure of that construct should behave?" (Levine et al., 2013).

Content validity: Content validity, also known as logical validity, refers to the extent to which a measure represents all facets of a given social construct. For example, a depression scale may lack content validity if it only assesses the affective dimension of depression but fails to take into account the behavioral dimension. Content validity is different from face validity, which refers not to what the test actually measures, but to what it superficially appears to measure. It requires the use of recognized subject matter experts to evaluate whether test items assess defined content and more rigorous statistical tests than does the assessment of face validity (Levine et al., 2013).

Core standards: The fundamental simulation education standards that have been developed by the Society for Simulation in Healthcare Certification Committee as a cooperative effort with input from other simulation societies and groups. The high level categories are (i) professional values and capabilities; (ii) knowledge of educational principles, practice, and methodology in simulation; (iii) implementing, assessing, and managing simulation-based education interventions; and (iv) scholarship—spirit of inquiry and teaching (SSH).

Critical thinking: A disciplined process that requires validation of data, including any assumptions that may influence thoughts and actions, and then careful reflection on the entire process while evaluating the effectiveness of what has been determined as the necessary action(s) to take. This process entails purposeful, goal-directed thinking and is based on scientific principles and methods (evidence) rather than assumptions or conjecture (Meakim et al., 2013).

Cueing: Information provided by instructors or designated participants in the simulation that helps the student progress through the simulation activity by providing information about the step the student is on or is approaching (SIRC).

Cut Suit: Product created by Strategic Operations, Inc. (STOPS) which developed the human worn partial task surgical simulator (aka "Cut Suit") that supports two separate training requirements; the first is for tactical combat casualty care (TCCC) and the second is as a surgical simulator. The Cut Suit used in realistic scenarios simulates the treatment of the three most common causes of preventable death on the battlefield, including hemorrhage from extremity wounds, tension pneumothorax, and airway compromise (Levine et al., 2013).

Debriefing: Activity that follows a simulation experience led by a facilitator wherein feedback is provided on the simulation participants' performance while positive aspects of the completed simulation are discussed and reflective thinking encouraged (SIRC).

DM: Diabetes mellitus.

DOB: Date of birth.

ECHO: Echocardiography, echocardiogram.

EEG: Electroencephalography or electroencephalograph.

Embedded participant: Also known as scenario guide, scenario role player, or confederate; the embedded participant is a role assigned in a simulation encounter to help guide the scenario. The guidance may be influential as positive, negative, or neutral or as a distractor, depending on the objective(s), the level of the participants, and the scenario. Although the embedded participant's role is part of the situation, the underlying purpose of the role may not be revealed to the participants in the scenario or simulation (Meakim et al., 2013).

ETOH: Ethyl alcohol.

Evidence-based: Educational materials or methods that have been proven through rigorous evaluation and research (SSH).

Experiential learning: The process of making meaning from direct experience. Simply put, experiential learning is learning from experience. The experience can be staged or left open. Experiential learning is learning through reflection on doing, which is often contrasted with rote or didactic learning (Levine et al., 2013).

Face validity: Face validity is the extent to which a test is subjectively viewed as covering the concept it purports to measure. It refers to the transparency or relevance of a test as they appear to test participants. Face validity assesses whether the test "looks valid" to the examinees who take it, the administrative personnel who decide on its use, and other technically untrained observers. In simulation, the first goal of the simulation modeler is to construct a model that appears reasonable on its face to model users and others who are knowledgeable about the real system being simulated (Levine et al., 2013).

Facilitation: Broadly used to describe any activity which makes tasks for others easy, or tasks that are assisted.

Feedback: Information given or dialogue between participants, facilitator, simulator, or peer with the intention of improving the understanding of concepts or aspects of performance (Meakim et al., 2013).

FHM: Fetal heart monitor.

FHR: Fetal heart rate.

Fidelity: Describes the level of realism associated with a particular simulation activity. It is not constrained to a certain type of simulation modality, and higher levels of fidelity are not required for a simulation to be successful. It is typically desirable to increase fidelity where reasonable, however (SSH).

Formative evaluation: Evaluation wherein the evaluator's focus is on the learner's progress toward goal achievement. A process for determining the competence of a person engaged in a healthcare activity for the purpose of providing constructive feedback for that person to improve (SIRC).

FSBS: Finger stick blood sugar.

Full body patient simulator: A realistic, full-body, wireless manikin which offers comprehensive clinical functionality to teach the core skills of airway, breathing, cardiac, and circulation management.

Full scale simulation: A device or scenario that allows simulation of tasks related to applicable learners for a given operational requirement. It is capable of simulating the operational environment (e.g., audio, visual, and tactile) to achieve maximum realism and training effectiveness (Levine et al., 2013).

Guided reflection: The process used by the facilitator during debriefing that reinforces the critical aspects of the experience and encourages insightful learning, allowing the participant to assimilate theory, practice, and research in order to influence future actions (Meakim et al., 2013).

Haptic: Refers to the sense of touch (from Greek haptikos ό="I fasten onto, I touch"). It is a tactile feedback technology which takes advantage of the sense of touch by applying forces, vibrations, or motions to the user. This mechanical stimulation can be used to assist in the creation of virtual objects in a computer simulation, to control such virtual objects, and to enhance the remote control of machines and devices (telerobotics). Haptic devices may incorporate tactile sensors that measure forces exerted by the user on the interface (Levine et al., 2013).

High fidelity simulator: This term is used to refer to a broad range of full-body manikins that have the ability to mimic, at a very high level, human body functions (SSH).

High-stakes assessment: A high-stakes assessment is one having important consequences for the test taker, and serves as the basis of a major decision. Passing is associated with important benefits, such as satisfaction of a licensure and/or certification requirement, or meeting a contingency for employment. Failing too has important consequences, such as being required to take remedial classes until the assessment can be passed, or being banned from practice within a certain discipline or domain. Thus, high-stakes assessment is one that (i) is a single, defined assessment, (ii) has clear distinction between those who pass and those who fail, and (iii) has direct consequences for passing or failing, for example, something is "at stake" (SSH).

HoTN: Hypotension.

HTN: Hypertension.

Human factors: The discipline or science of studying the interaction between humans and systems and technology. The term covers all biomedical and psychological considerations (VHA SimLearn, 2015).

Hx: History, history of.

H&P: History and physical.

Hybrid simulation: Integrating different types of simulation across different dimensions of applications, purposes, and target populations and assessing the impact or benefit of simulation-based training across the various dimensions (Gaba, 2004).

In situ/In-Situ/In-situ: Describes an educational activity that takes place in the actual patient care area/setting in which the healthcare providers would normally function. This does not include a setting that is "made" to look like a work area (SSH).

Interprofessional education: When two or more professionals learn about, from, and with each other to enable effective collaboration and improve health outcomes (Meakim et al., 2013).

IV: Intravenous.

Laparoscopy: Also called minimally invasive surgery (MIS), bandaid surgery, or keyhole surgery and is a modern surgical technique in which operations in the abdomen are performed through small incisions (usually 0.5–1.5 cm) as opposed to the larger incisions needed in laparotomy. The key element in laparoscopic surgery is the use of a laparoscope. There are two types: (1) a telescopic rod lens system that is usually connected to a video camera (single chip or three chip) or (2) a digital laparoscope where the charge-coupled device is placed at the end of the laparoscope, eliminating the rod lens system. Also attached is a fiber-optic cable system connected to a "cold" light source (halogen or xenon), to illuminate the operative field, inserted through a 5 or 10 mm cannula or trocar to view the operative field. The abdomen is usually insufflated, or essentially blown up like a balloon, with carbon dioxide gas. This elevates the abdominal wall above the internal organs like a dome to create a working and viewing space. CO_2 is used because it is common to the human body and can be absorbed by tissue and removed by the respiratory system. It is also non-flammable, which is important because electrosurgical devices are commonly used in laparoscopic procedures (Levine et al., 2013).

LP: Lumbar puncture.

Manikin/Mannikin/Mannequin/Manakin (other): These are part-or-full-body simulators that can have varying levels of function and fidelity. There is usually additional descriptive terminology that is added to allow for understanding of what type of manikin is being described (SSH).

Microsimulation: Synonym for laptop or web-based simulation (VHA SimLEARN, 2015). Retrieved from http://www.simlearn.va.gov/SIMLEARN/NAV_Glossary_SimLEARN.asp.

Mixed simulation (mixed methods simulation): The use of a variety of different types of simulations simultaneously. This is different from hybrid simulation in that it is not characterized by the use of one type of simulation to enhance another, but rather the use of multiple types of simulation as part of the overall educational activity (SSH).

Modality: A term used to refer to the type(s) of simulation being used as part of the educational activity. (e.g., task trainers, manikin-based, standardized/simulated patients, computer-based, virtual reality, and hybrid (SSH).

Modeling and simulation (M&S): The use of models (e.g., emulators, prototypes, simulators, and stimulators) either statically or over time to develop data as a basis for making managerial or technical decisions (Palaganas et al., 2015).

Moulage: A French term to mean (i) a mold, as of a footprint, made for use in a criminal investigation and (ii) the making of such a mold or cast, as with plaster of Paris. For simulation it has meant to mean the makeup and molds applied to actors or mannequins used to portray lesions, skin findings, and bleeding and traumatized areas (Levine et al., 2013).

MRSA: Methicillin-resistant staphylococcus aureus.

MVC: Motor vehicle collision.

NG: Nasogastric.

NKA: No known allergies.

Nontechnical skills: Behavioral skills which can be categorized as either (i) skills of dynamic decision-making (e.g., anticipation and planning, use of cognitive aids, avoiding fixation errors) or (ii) skills of teamwork and team management (e.g., workload distribution, communication, and/or role clarity) (VHA SimLEARN, 2015). Retrieved from http://www.simlearn.va.gov/SIMLEARN/NAV_Glossary_SimLEARN.asp.

Objective: Statement(s) of specific measurable results that participant(s) is expected to achieve during a simulation-based learning experience (Meakim et al., 2013).

OSCE (pronounced "Ahss-Kee"), aka Objective Structured Clinical Examination: The OSCE is a station or series of stations designed to assess performance competency in individual clinical or other professional skills. Stations are carefully structured and designed to be easily reproducible. Learners are evaluated via direct observation, checklists, learner presentation or written follow-up exercises. The examinations are generally summative but may involve feedback. Stations tend to be short, typically 5–10 minutes, but can be longer (Meakim et al., 2013).

On-the-fly approach: The term simply connotes being in a mobile or fluid situation. *Webster's New World Dictionary* states that the term probably originated with bird hunting and shooting birds on the fly (rather than on the ground). The dictionary says simply "in flight" and adds a colloquial meaning of "in a hurry." In relation to computer technology, "on the fly" describes activities that develop or occur dynamically rather than as the result of something that is statically predefined.

Operator-driven approach: Relying on direct control by the operator of all the clinical data and features, sometimes augmented by software "scripts" to automate certain stereotyped responses in well-defined clinical situations (VHA SimLEARN, 2015). Retrieved from http://www.simlearn.va.gov/SIMLEARN/NAV_Glossary_ SimLEARN.asp.

Prebriefing/briefing: An information or orientation session held prior to the start of a simulation-based learning experience in which instructions or preparatory information is given to the participants. The purpose of the prebriefing or briefing is to set the stage for a scenario and assist participants in achieving scenario objectives. Suggested activities in a prebriefing or briefing include an orientation to the equipment, environment, mannequin, roles, time allotment, objectives, and patient situation (Meakim et al., 2013).

Pre-programmed (or programmed) scenario: Scenarios that include a combination of *automated* physiological and/or pathophysiological model(s) of the medical condition and a complex decision-making tree that reflect(s) the patient's response(s) to the various clinical/medical interventions that lead to any number of possible clinical outcomes. The programming of the scenario is represented by a proprietary file, or files, unique to a particular manufacturer. Some companies and institutions are commissioning, developing, marketing and selling such files and associated supplemental educational and implementation materials. Programmed scenarios, whether purchased, or programmed by a simulation program's own educators and/operations specialists are subjected to a rigorous validation process to ensure accuracy and alignment with best practices specific to the objectives of the scenario design. Additional benefits of programmed scenarios is the ability to standardize scenario participant experiences and to allow the operator and/or facilitator to focus on observed participant interactions during the scenario. For the most part "pre-preprogrammed" and "programmed" terms are used interchangeably, but some have associated "pre-programmed" with automated outcomes associated with physiological modeling and other built-in capabilities.

PRN: Pro re nata—as needed.

Problem-based learning: Small group learning with a facilitator where the students access and engage as a group with the VP (virtual patient) case (VHA SimLEARN, 2015). Retrieved from http://www.simlearn.va.gov/SIMLEARN/NAV_Glossary_SimLEARN.asp.

Prompt: A cue given to a participant in a scenario (Meakim et al., 2013).

QSEN: The Quality and Safety Education for Nurses (QSEN) project began in 2005 and was funded by the Robert Wood Johnson Foundation (RWJF). The overall goal of QSEN has been to address the challenge of preparing future nurses with the knowledge, skills, and attitudes (KSA) necessary to continuously improve the quality and safety of the healthcare systems in which they work (Meakim et al., 2013).

Readback: An order is given; it is written down and read back. It is then acknowledged by giver as correct (VHA SimLEARN, 2015).

Reliability: The extent to which a measure is consistent across repeated tests and includes test-retest reliability correlation of tests applied more than once to same subjects, internal consistency correlation of subsets of scores measuring same construct, and inter-rater reliability degree of agreement between multiple raters of same test subjects (VHA SimLEARN, 2015).

Remote feedback: Uses all the distant interconnection technology to bring together participants, observers, and instructors for a shared experience, without each and every one of them actually bringing themselves to a common observation/debriefing room (VHA SimLEARN, 2015).

RR: Respiratory rate.

SBAR: Acronym for "situation," "background," "assessment," and "recommendation." It allows a clinical team member to easily and quickly describe the clinical presentation of a patient and make a recommendation for future action. It is a component of effective communication between one healthcare provider and another (VHA SimLEARN, 2015).

Simulated patient, Standardized patient: In healthcare, is an individual who is trained to act as a real patient in order to simulate a set of symptoms or problems. Simulated patients have been successfully used in medical education, nursing education, evaluation, and research. Recent technology has allowed for the simulated patient to exist as a mannequin, robot, or Web-or computer-based avatar (Levine et al., 2013).

Simulation: Is the imitation of the operation of a real-world process or system over time. The act of simulating something first requires that a model be developed; this model represents the key characteristics or behaviors of the selected physical or abstract system or process. The model represents the system itself, whereas the simulation represents the operation of the system over time. Simulation is used in many contexts, such as simulation of technology for performance optimization, safety engineering, testing, training, education, and video games. Training simulators include flight simulators for training aircraft pilots to provide them with a lifelike experience. Simulation is also used with scientific modeling of natural systems or human systems to gain insight into their functioning. Simulation can be used to show the eventual real effects of alternative conditions and courses of action. Simulation is also used when the real system cannot be engaged, because it may not be accessible, or it may be dangerous or unacceptable to engage, or it is being designed but not yet built, or it may simply not exist (Levine et al., 2013).

Simulation fidelity: Refers to the simulation—how the simulator is used in context to represent a patient care situation—rather than to the simulator device itself (VHA SimLEARN, 2015).

Simulation guideline: Generally to follow the critical thinking process of assessment, diagnosis, planning, intervening, and evaluation of care for a patient in a short time frame. Each scenario has a patient introduction, contact with the patient, and then time to debrief about the care. There are learning objectives: (i) apply critical thinking in the care of an adult client experiencing and adapting to complex, multi-system dysfunctions and (ii) apply scientific, theoretical knowledge and advanced clinical skills to provide safe and competent holistic nursing care of the medical-surgical client within professional standards of practice. There are also learning outcomes: (i) prioritize critical clinical/medical actions based on analysis of data from assessing the patient, chart, and report given, (ii) identify roles of the members of the team, (iii) interpret the diagnostic information, (iv) compare and contrast the various medications used for the patient, (v) demonstrate accurate documentation/communication of the clinical plan of care, (vi) apply principles of holistic care to address patient care needs, (vii) demonstrate participation as a healthcare team member undergoing crisis management of a critical patient, (viii) demonstrate coordination of the healthcare team undergoing crisis management of a critical patient, and (ix) evaluate and discuss patient care outcomes.

Simulation standard: Refers to a model, example, or rule for the measure of quantity, weight, extent, value, or quality, established by authority, custom, or general consent. It is also defined as a criterion, gauge, or yardstick by which judgments or decisions may be made. A meaningful standard should offer a realistic prospect of determining whether or not one actually meets it (VHA SimLEARN, 2015).

Simulation validity: The degree to which simulation accurately measures the intended concept of interest (Meakim et al., 2013).

SOB: Shortness of breath.

Standardized patient: A simulated patient, standardized patient, or sample patient (SP) (also known as a patient instructor), in healthcare, is an individual who is trained to act as a real patient in order to simulate a set of symptoms or problems. Simulated patients have been successfully used in medical education, nursing education, evaluation, and research (Levine et al., 2013).

Summative assessment (summative evaluation): A process for determining the competence of a person engaged in a healthcare activity for the purpose of certifying with reasonable certainty that they are able to perform that activity in practice (SSH).

Summative evaluation: Evaluation at the end of a time period, in which participants are provided with feedback about their achievement of outcome criteria; a process for determining the competence of a participant engaged in an activity. The assessment of achievement of outcome criteria may be associated with an assigned grade, demonstration of competency, merit pay, promotion, or certification (Meakim et al., 2013).

Summative feedback: Information provided by a facilitator regarding aspects of performance that are associated with the assignment of a grade, demonstration of competency, merit pay, promotion, or certification. It usually involves setting of expectations and standards; systematically gathering, analyzing, and interpreting evidence; and using resulting information to document, explain, or improve performance (Meakim et al., 2013).

Task fixation: In medicine, task fixation results from a physician, in a crisis situation, getting fixated on a single procedure, when instead, he/she should team lead and delegate tasks to those who are qualified to perform the tasks at hand. In simulation, task fixation can occur when the student is not observant of the simulation as a whole, and instead begins to focus on a single task instead of calling for assistance.

Technical skills: The actual performance of patient care treatment (VHA SimLEARN, 2015).

TPR: Temperature, pulse, respiration.

UTI: Urinary tract infection.

Validity: Translational outcomes. Educational effects measured at increasingly distal levels beginning in the classroom or simulation laboratory and moving downstream to improved and safer patient care practices, better patient outcomes, and collateral educational effects, such as cost savings, skills retention, and systematic educational and patient care improvements (McGaghie, Issenberg, Barsuk, & Wayne, 2014).

Virtual reality simulations: The simulated environment can be similar to the real world in order to create a lifelike experience—for example, in simulations for pilot or combat training—or it can differ significantly from reality, such as in VR games. In practice, it is currently very difficult to create a high fidelity virtual reality experience, due largely to technical limitations on processing power, image resolution, and communication bandwidth; however, the technology's proponents hope that such limitations will be overcome as processor, imaging, and data communication technologies become more powerful and cost effective over time (Levine et al., 2013).

REFERENCES

Gaba, D. M. (2004). The future vision of simulation in health care. *Quality and Safety in Health Care, 13,* i2–i10. doi:10.1136/qshc.2004.009878

Gaba, D. M., Howard, S. K., Flanagan, B., Smith, B. E., Fish, K. J., & Botney, R. (1998). Assessment of clinical performance during simulated crises using both technical and behavioral ratings. *Anesthesiology, 89*(1), 8–18.

Levine, A. I., DeMaria, S., & Schwartz, A. D. (Eds.). (2013). *Comprehensive textbook of healthcare simulation.* New York, NY: Springer.

McGaghie, W. C., Issenberg, S. B., Barsuk, J. H., & Wayne, D. B. (2014). A critical review of simulation-based mastery learning with translational outcomes. *Medical Education, 48,* 375–385.

Meakim, C., Boese, T., Decker, S., Franklin, A., Gloe, D., Lioce, L., … Borum, J. C. (2013). Standards of best practice: Simulation. Standard 1: Terminology. *Clinical Simulation in Nursing, 9,* S3–11.

Palaganas, J. C., Maxworthy, J. C., Epps, C. A., & Mancini, M. E. (Eds.). (2015). *Defining excellence in simulation programs.* Philadelphia, PA: Society for Simulation in Healthcare/ Lippincott Wolters, Kluwer.

Society for Simulation in Healthcare (SSH). (2015). Appendix III: Certification terminology. *SSH certified healthcare simulation operations specialist handbook.* Retrieved from http:// www.ssih.org/Portals/48/Certification/CHSOS_Docs/CHSOS%20Handbook.pdf

VHA SimLEARN. (2015). *Clinical simulation and resuscitation glossary of training terms.* Retrieved from http://www.simlearn.va.gov/SIMLEARN/NAV_Glossary_SimLEARN.asp

APPENDIX 2

SIMULATION OPERATIONS SPECIALISTS JOB DESCRIPTIONS EXEMPLARS

Laura T. Gantt

East Carolina University College of Nursing, Greenville, NC, USA

Sample Position Description
Hospital Setting
Simulation Specialist

Department: Simulation and Clinical Skills
Schedule: Full-time FTE 0.9–1.0
Shift: AM
Hours: 8
Job Details:
Job Summary:

Responsible for the installation, maintenance, and general operation of high technology patient simulators, lower technology task trainers, clinical equipment, and related multimedia peripherals used in the training of healthcare professionals from all specialties. Will demonstrate and/or teach technical aspects of operating the simulators and related equipment to center staff, faculty members, and others when appropriate. Will assist educators with the development of customized simulation activities which enhance learning through the incorporation of appropriate simulation technologies. Will also assist with simulation-related research efforts as designated.

All team members are expected to be knowledgeable and compliant with Palmetto Health's values of compassion, dignity, excellence, integrity, and teamwork.

Healthcare Simulation: A Guide for Operations Specialists, First Edition.
Edited by Laura T. Gantt and H. Michael Young.
© 2016 John Wiley & Sons, Inc. Published 2016 by John Wiley & Sons, Inc.

Responsibilities:

Communicate in a positive, professional manner with co-workers, faculty instructors, students, and other users of the simulation center. This includes both written and verbal communication.

Assist faculty and other staff of the simulation center in the operational aspects of simulation.

Assist with special projects or initiatives as required.

Design, develop, implement, and evaluate scenarios and educational material in collaboration with faculty, simulation center staff, and other users of the simulation center.

Provide faculty instructors with instructional tools and technical or administrative support to carry out simulation sessions. This includes setting up the simulator, the rooms, and appropriate audio-video components for each session, and preparing educational material for the activity as directed.

Understand the use and operation of different simulator technologies ranging from partial task trainers to high fidelity patient simulators to virtual reality simulators.

Interface with the equipment manufacturers regarding equipment troubleshooting and systems problems as well as periodic upgrades; maintain record of repairs.

Perform all required equipment maintenance and troubleshooting while actively maintaining proficiency in existing and emerging technologies, including basic theory, design, and implementation.

Perform and synthesize literature searches, analyze and summarize relevant material, and maintain reference library of simulation articles.

Participate in technical training as necessary; attend conferences to stay current with simulation technologies and education modalities.

Generate innovative approaches for technology improvement and integration into healthcare education.

Requirements:

Education: Minimum of 2 years of college in clinical healthcare field (nursing preferred). Four years college preferred. Some experience may be accepted as substitute.

Experience: 4–6 years in a related field.

License, Registry, or Certification Required: RN, EMT, or Paramedic preferred; BLS or BCLS required. Valid SC driver's license and an acceptable 3 year motor vehicle record as defined by the Acceptable Motor Vehicle Record Chart are required since this job requires operation of a Palmetto Health vehicle. Employee will be expected to adhere to the Palmetto Health Driver Safety Policy and specific department driving policies and must pass driver training.

Special Training: Flexibility and service orientation are required. Must be able to vary schedule and to work overtime, occasionally with minimal notice, as client activities dictate. Knowledge of medical terminology is required. Proficiency navigation a must. Operation and maintenance of high technology, electronic human patient simulators, and low tech task trainers or an aptitude to learn use and maintenance of specialized simulation and clinical equipment.

EEO/AA

WEBSITE

Retrieved from https://www.healthcaresource.com/palmetto/index.cfm
Sample Job Description and Evaluation
Tech Support Technician
Academic Setting

Working Title: Tech Support Technician
Classification Title: Tech Support Technician
Division: Health Sciences
Department: HS Nurs Administration

CORE WORK VALUES

Customer Service

- Identifies who their internal and external customers are.
- Determines the needs of internal and external customers and is attentive to those needs.
- Treats all customers in a professional, respectful, friendly, and courteous manner.
- Resolves customer concerns.
- Anticipates and provides what customers need to enhance their experience.
- Fully uses available resources, including technology, to enhance customer service.
- Responds to phone/email messages, uses "out of office" message for email and phone, as appropriate, as specified within departmental guidelines.
- Answers phone calls when possible instead of allowing them to go into voice mail on a routine basis.

Compliance

- Complies with any university- and/or departmental-specific programs, related policies and procedures, guidelines, expectations, etc. (including performance and conduct) as well as standards of safety, accreditation, and other regulations.
- Identifies and reports in good faith potential incidents of noncompliance to supervisor or other appropriate officer.

Diversity

- Is willing to explore and overcome own biases.
- Is open to different ideas and approaches.
- Learns about characteristics, values, and beliefs that are different from one's own.
- Acknowledges and respects different customs and values in meeting customer needs.
- Is courteous and nonjudgmental when interacting with others.
- Respects, appreciates, and values all employees as individuals.

Excellence

- Evaluates current processes and develops alternatives to improve processes and work outcomes while decreasing costs.
- Recognizes that all ideas and approaches have value.
- Encourages the development of new ideas.
- Accepts responsibility for developing self and proactively initiates development opportunities.
- Seeks, accepts, and acts on feedback from supervisors, peers, and customers.
- Supports continuous individual and organizational assessment and improvement.
- Sets high, realistic goals for him/herself.

Respect and Honesty

- Recognizes the impact of his/her behavior on others.
- Is responsible for his/her behavior toward others.
- Expresses concerns about work issues and works constructively to create a resolution.
- Is sensitive to the personal concerns and beliefs of others.
- Interacts in an honest manner with all people inside and outside of the system.
- Addresses any dishonest or unethical behavior, both upwards and peer-to-peer.
- Admits, corrects, and learns from mistakes.
- Acts in a compassionate manner with everyone.

Communication

- Promotes an environment that supports open communication.
- Provides appropriate information to others in a respectful and helpful manner.
- Communicates with all customers in a professional manner.

Dependability

- Consistently adheres to assigned work schedule.
- Appropriately requests leave using departmental guidelines for calling out of work.
- Maintains positive leave balances.
- Ensures work is completed timely and appropriately.
- Follows up appropriately and as necessary.

SUPERVISOR/MANAGERIAL CORE WORK VALUES

Human Resources Management

- Approves work schedules and oversees daily operations.
- Participates in the hiring process.

- Responsible for new staff orientation.
- Conducts all performance appraisals/competency assessments in a timely manner in accordance with policy.
- Participates in personnel coaching, counseling, and implements performance improvement/career development plans as needed.
- Promotes a positive, motivating environment support of staff retention.
- Manages staff behavior and timely resolves issues, individually and within the department.

Leadership

- Demonstrates commitment to university and organizational values.
- Demonstrates appreciation of workplace diversity.
- Exhibits professionalism in evaluating and recognizing staff performance and promotes staff development.
- Establishes clear two-way communication with all staff to ensure accountability and understanding of pertinent issues.
- Meets regularly with staff to communicate organizational and departmental priorities.
- Functions as a liaison between individuals and groups.

Budget/Financial Management

- Operates department/unit within allocated budget, as appropriate.
- Seeks additional resources for funding, as appropriate.

TECHNICAL EXPERTISE

Technical equipment (hardware and software) is central to the department's ability to provide realistic lab experiences for students. The person in this position will:

- Assist with planning, implementation, teaching, and utilization of clinical information systems and technical laboratory equipment.
- Provide technical expertise and leadership in simulation technologies, including programming and running the technical component of healthcare simulation scenarios.
- Provide full multimedia support, including capture, editing, and delivery of lab sessions and healthcare scenarios.
- Prepare and operate technical equipment for labs and classroom activities.
- Assist with technical configuration in preparing equipment and materials for scheduled lab activities, including lab exercises and demonstrations.
- Provide technical support to faculty and staff as they work with students in the lab.
- Install, configure, and maintain software to support labs activities.

TRAINING

Proper utilization of technical equipment is essential to successful laboratory clinical training. A key role of this position is to assist with the implementation and with the understanding of implementation of the laboratory technical tools. The person in this position will:

- Assist in the development of online training and instructional materials for nursing instructors and students.
- Provide technical advice and assistance during lab practical classes.
- Participate in scheduled in-service activities.
- Advise instructors on lab technical materials and consult on how best to implement those materials to achieve course goals.

COLLABORATION/COMMUNICATION

An important component for a successful clinical laboratory program is effective communication, not only internally among faculty and clinical lab sections, but also externally, with departments and schools within the university, and also with other universities and entities throughout the healthcare community. The person in this position will:

- Develop and maintain web materials to support lab activities.
- Represent the department in special technology projects within the college.
- Communicate professionally with students, staff, and faculty to achieve the goals of the department in providing a desirable learning environment and in assuring the effective operation of the lab.
- Work collaboratively with other departments to support interdisciplinary student training and research.
- Support scholarly activities, including research, student and faculty surveys, presentations and quality improvement projects.
- Provide public relations and consultation opportunities for other schools and entities as requested.

TECHNOLOGY EVALUATION

The technology associated with healthcare simulation is evolving rapidly. To maintain excellence in clinical laboratory training, it is imperative to periodically evaluate technology currently in use, and to be aware of innovations and new technology in the field. The person in this position will:

- Assist in the evaluation of current technologies used by the department, including hardware, software, and their implementations and methodologies of deployment.
- Assist in the evaluation of new clinical laboratory equipment.
- Assist in the evaluation of new clinical laboratory software.

NC 12247
OSP 6/2004

TECHNOLOGY SUPPORT TECHNICIAN

DESCRIPTION OF WORK:

This is a technical work in providing consultation, support, and/or training to clients of computer or other information technology-based systems. Employees are located throughout the state at agencies and universities. Employees provide basic support of hardware, applications, operating systems, and networking. This level requires a basic knowledge and understanding of a wide variety of technologies to effectively support clients' technical needs. Employees at this level are not usually involved in application development, system integration, or network design/analysis.

Employees interact with a broad range of clients requiring strong communication skills and ability to use a variety of technical resources for providing technical support. Employees at this level may provide routine support for a broad range of information-related technologies, or may provide in-depth support for a narrowly defined area of technology. Employees refer complex technical problems or questions to a higher-level technology support analyst and/or technology support specialist.

EXAMPLES OF COMPETENCIES:

CONTRIBUTING:

- **Planning and Organizing:** Ability to work independently on routine /noncomplex tasks.
- **Project Management:** Ability to participate as a productive project team member by completing assigned routine tasks.
- **Technical Knowledge:** Understanding of basic troubleshooting techniques and principles.
- **Technical Solution Development:** Knowledge of and may serve as a technical resource for basic solutions to clients.
- **Technical Support:** Ability to solicit relevant information from client in order to sufficiently describe nonroutine problems to technical expert and effectively communicate solution to client.
- **Consultancy Skills:** Ability to determine client needs and effectively communicate back to technical experts.

JOURNEY

- **Planning and Organizing:** Ability to organize and follow complex and/or detailed technical procedures.
- **Project Management:** Ability to participate as a project team member and make recommendations for routine problem solutions.
- **Technical Knowledge:** Ability to apply a broad working knowledge in a specialty area within a work unit.
- **Technical Solution Development:** Ability to identify and understand reoccurring problems and recommend solutions.
- **Technical Support:** Ability to independently resolve routine and some nonroutine problems through standard troubleshooting procedures. Able to perform routine diagnostics and/or configurations on assigned software and/or hardware according to standard operating procedures.
- **Consultancy Skills:** Ability to communicate and consult with clients and higher-level analysts to resolve technical problems.

ADVANCED

- **Planning and Organizing:** Ability to lead ad hoc work groups to analyze problems, develop solutions, and communicate solutions effectively. Ability to identify need for training in new technology or for reoccurring problems, either technical or procedural.
- **Project Management:** Ability to participate on a project team as an expert in a specialty area or work.
- **Technical Knowledge:** Significant knowledge in a technical specialty area. Ability to serve as a technical resource for other technicians, inclusive of training.
- **Technical Solution Development:** Ability to lead or guide journey level technician with technical solutions.

Ability to resolve complex problems within a work area.

- **Technical Support:** Ability to identify trends and make suggestions for technical modifications to prevent future problems.
- **Consultancy Skills:** Ability to communicate and consult with clients and higher-level specialists and analysts to resolve advanced technical problems and ensure customer satisfaction.

MINIMUM TRAINING AND EXPERIENCE:

High school diploma or equivalency and 1 year of experience in the field of technology related to the area of assignment; or equivalent combination of training and experience.

All degrees must be received from appropriately accredited institutions.

Special Note: This is a generalized representation of positions in this class and is not intended to reflect essential functions per ADA. Examples of competencies are typical of the majority of positions, but may not be applicable to all positions.

Class Spec Form—Updated 7/02

APPENDIX 3

CONNECTIONS

Image of Connection(s)	Description
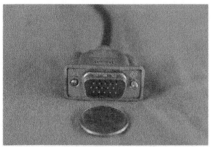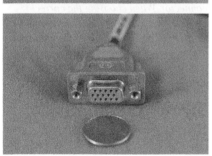	Video Graphics Array (VGA) is a 15-pin connector that has been used since the late 1980s. VGA only supports video, not audio like some of the other connectors shown. VGA transmits analog video only. *Example: There are several simulation manikins that use a VGA cable to connect a vital sign monitor. An external monitor is connected to the control computer and acts as an extended display that simulates a vital sign monitor one would find in clinical environment.*

(*continued*)

Image of Connection(s)	Description

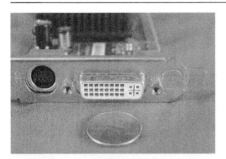

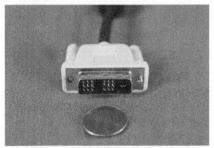

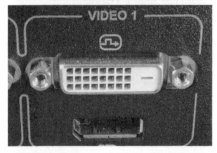

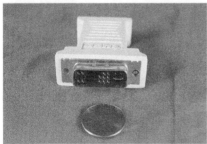

Digital Visual Interface (DVI) is a digital video connection that can also transmit analog video signal. There are three main different versions: DVI-D, DVI-A, and DVI-I. DVI-D stands for digital only; DVI-A, for analog only; and DVI-I, for *Integrated*, meaning digital and analog signals are combined. DVI connectors are typically white and are commonly found on computers. Note the difference between the connectors shown in the picture on the left. DVI-A and DVI-I utilize the four prongs on the right of the connector (surrounding the long flat prong) to transmit analog video.

Example: Some devices use DVI-D connectors and have no analog signal throughput. Therefore, trying to connect a DVI-A or DVI-I connector to a device that only accepts DVI-D may be impossible since the device with a DVI-D connection does not have holes to accommodate the four prongs that are included on a DVI-A or DVI-D connector. When choosing the correct DVI cable, it is important to determine the needed and accepted connectors that are used on the devices to be connected.

Image of Connection(s)	Description
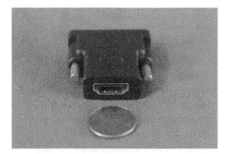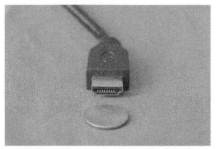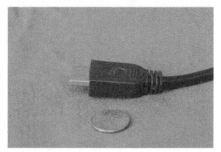	High-Definition Multimedia Interface (HDMI) is an interface for video and audio that is quickly replacing analog communications. HDMI transmits digital video and audio and can also transmit other information to help control devices connected via HDMI. Many output devices such as televisions, projectors, and monitors accept HDMI. Professional and consumer electronics rely on HDMI connectors when digital video is needed. HDMI technology is closely related to DVI connections and can typically be converted to/from DVI with no loss of definition. Just as with any digital transmission, an operations specialist would not be able to connect analog devices with HDMI connections without the use of a DAC, ADC, *video scaler*, or similar device.
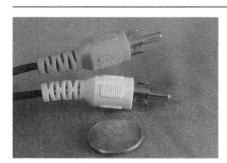	RCA connectors are coaxial-type connectors able to transmit video or audio signals. RCA connectors have been around since the 1940s and are still popular in a variety of applications. Since these cables are coaxial, they have two contacts, which limits them in the amount of information they can transmit. These cables are relatively simple and easy to use, making them cost-effective and popular in consumer electronics. These connections are found on many video output and input devices along with audio output and input devices. Digital audio can be transmitted via RCA connectors following an adapted version of RCA technology.

(continued)

Image of Connection(s)	Description
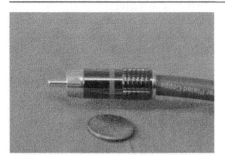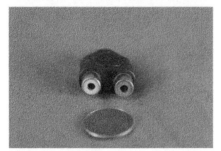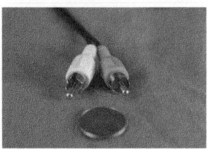	With so many uses for RCA connections, it is helpful to keep in mind that most RCA connectors follow a color scheme to indicate the purpose of a connection (i.e., red and white for right and left audio, respectively, and yellow for composite video). An Internet search for RCA connector color schemes would deliver an abundance of helpful information.
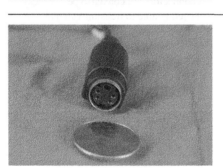	S-Video connectors transmit analog video typically in standard resolution. This technology is quickly being replaced with other technologies but can still be found on many displays and projectors.

Image of Connection(s)	Description
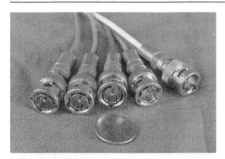 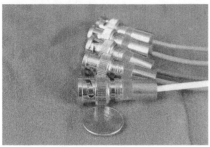	BNC connectors are very similar to RCA connectors but are typically found in permanent or professional installations. These connectors are coaxial, offering two contacts, and have a locking mechanism that makes it easy to ensure they stay in place.
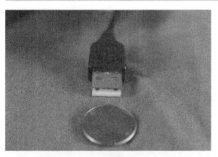 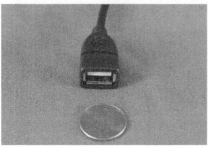	Universal Serial Bus (USB) connections are essentially serial connections that have been made smaller and faster. These connections serve as data connections (e.g., external storage or devices) for computers. These external devices may sometimes be cameras, such as webcams, or audio devices such as headphones or microphones. USB connections are not commonly used to send *uncompressed* or analog audio signal like a microphone cable but may transmit digital audio to a device and therefore essentially serve as a digital audio connection. The same is true with video where the cable is not passing uncompressed or analog video but may be used to transmit digital video data and therefore serve as a digital video connection.

(*continued*)

Image of Connection(s)	Description
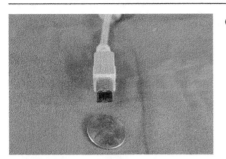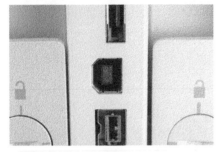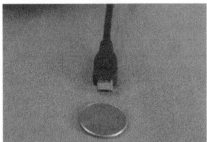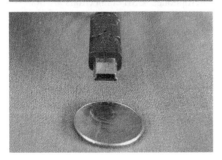	Common variations of USB connectors include USB standard-A plug and standard-A receptacle, standard-B, and mini-B. USB standard-A receptacles are commonly found in computers designed to accept USB standard-A plugs such as those on USB headsets or storage drives. Standard-B plugs generally plug into devices such printers that would have a standard-B receptacle. Mini-B plugs are common connectors for devices such as cameras that have less space to accommodate larger connections.

Image of Connection(s)	Description
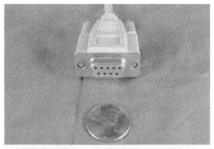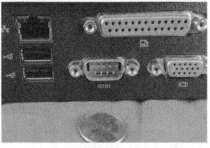	Serial (or RS-232) is a communication interface (or *COM port*) that is able to transfer data. RS-232 connections have been used since the 1950s and use a 9-pin connector (technically named DE-9). This cable is being superseded by USB technology for use with many devices but can still be found on some hardware that is configured by a computer (e.g., routers or professional audio processing units). These cables can connect devices to be controlled by computers but do not typically transmit audio or video. Several popular devices found in the simulation environment have historically utilized this type of connector. It is helpful to know that due to the physical nature of these cables, cables with lengths over 15 meters can cause reliability issues.
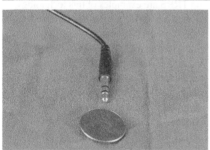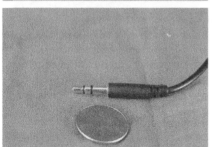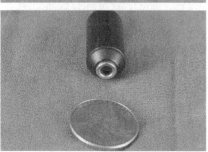	3.5 mm (1/8 inch [⅛″]) connectors are commonly found in consumer electronics as headphone jacks. These connectors are used on computers as headphones and microphone jacks. Typically, these connectors offer stereo audio signals and do not transmit video. *Example: Several popular manikins utilize the control computer's headphone jack as a way to transmit audio of recorded voice to speaker or amplifier to emulate the voice of a patient.* *There are other simulators that use the computer's 3.5 mm microphone input to allow an operator to speak through the manikin speakers so it sounds as though the patient were speaking.*

(*continued*)

Image of Connection(s)	Description
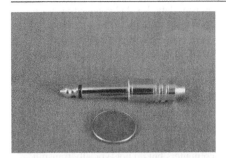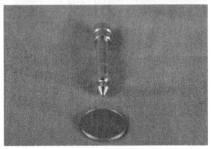	¼″ plugs (quarter-inch connectors) are commonly used to transmit analog audio. Some applications of this type of connector would include electronic instruments and various audio sources. Sometimes referred to as *patch cables* or, in its stereo or *balanced* form, tip–ring–sleeve (TRS) cables, these connectors are used in a wide variety of applications. Early versions of this included *phone cables* that have ¼″ connectors and were used on phone switchboards. TRS and tip–ring–ring–sleeve (TRRS) versions increase the availability of contacts on the connectors. Tip–sleeve (TS, or standard mono) connectors have two contacts, allowing one audio signal. TRS and TRRS are examples of this technology adapted to provide greater performance. This adapted technology is found in 3.5 mm connectors as well. TRS cables allow for two signals (commonly used for stereo headphones), whereas TRRS cables, with four contacts, allow three signals (commonly found in stereo headphones with the third signal used for microphone, such as Apple iPhone™ headphones).
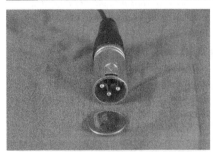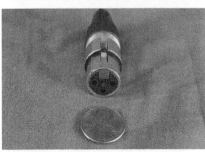	XLR connectors are common connectors used for audio equipment. Typically consisting of three pins/connectors, XLR connections are a reliable way to transmit a single *balanced* analog audio signal. The male and female connectors are able to latch, avoiding accidental unplugging. There are many variations of the connector, also known as a *Cannon plug* that may have fewer or more connectors. Some manufacturers of lighting and audio equipment may adopt a less common version of this connector to achieve a certain connection that requires four, five, or more contacts; these connections can also be used for the transfer of power.

Image of Connection(s)	Description

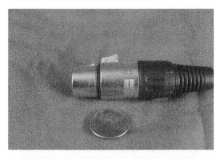

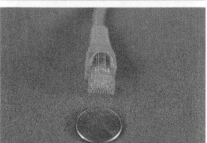

In the simulation environment, the XRL connector is commonly found on microphones and audio mixers. These connectors are relatively easy to terminate and can be "jumped" (use an additional cable to act as an extension). This, with low cost and ready availability, makes these connectors very common in any technical application involving audio.

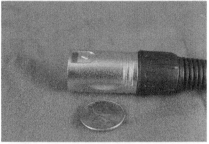

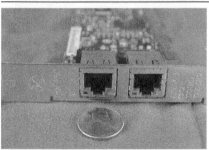

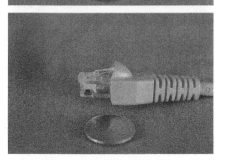

Ethernet connections are a wiring technology primarily used in networking. Most connections consist of a Cat 5, Cat 5e, or Cat 6 cable terminated with a RJ45 connector (shown here). There are eight contacts. These cables can be terminated easily, their cost is relatively low, they provide high networking speeds, and they can be run 100 meters with minimal performance loss. These connectors are generally used to connect a computer NIC to a LAN though there are many applications of Ethernet cables that do not involve networking. One example would be an active USB extension that utilizes adaptors on the ends of an Ethernet cable to transmit USB signal.

(*continued*)

Image of Connection(s)	Description
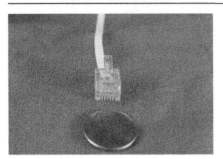	RJ11 is the commonly recognized connector for a phone jack. This connector is becoming less popular with the evolution of Ethernet (RJ45) technology but is still seen on phones and some computer modems.

APPENDIX 4

FILE FORMATS

EVAN J. BARTLEY

ECU College of Nursing, Greenville, NC, USA

Common file extensions utilized in office as well as in simulation environments.

Extension	File-Type Name	Description
.doc, .docx	Microsoft Word Document	This file is a document that is generally created and edited by Microsoft Word™, although there are third party applications that can generate and edit this type of file.
.xls, .xlsx	Microsoft Excel Spreadsheet	This file is a spreadsheet (or a book of spreadsheets) used by Microsoft Excel™. There are third party applications that can modify excel spreadsheets.
.pdf	Portable Document Format	This is a document file that can be read with a free application. Originally a proprietary platform developed by Adobe(R), in 2008, the PDF architecture became an open standard. PDFs can be generated with various applications as a way to deliver documents to users that may not have access to expensive software. PDFs are widely used as a way to distribute documentation online; this file is not easily manipulated and allows a feature to electronically sign a document.

(continued)

Healthcare Simulation: A Guide for Operations Specialists, First Edition.
Edited by Laura T. Gantt and H. Michael Young.
© 2016 John Wiley & Sons, Inc. Published 2016 by John Wiley & Sons, Inc.

Extension	File-Type Name	Description
.jpg .png .gif .tiff	Various image files	These are image files. JPG and GIF utilize common compression formats for images that retain decent quality without taking up too much space. PNG files are web-friendly files that can be displayed with most internet browsers. Typically, TIFF image files are uncompressed image information files.
.wav .aiff. mp3	Various audio files	These audio files are common on both MAC and IBM-PC computers. WAV and AIFF files are typically uncompressed audio files; WAV files can be found on most audio CDs. MP3 is one of many compressed audio formats. Compressed audio, like images, will require less disk space but at the sacrifice of definition.
.avi .wmv .mov .m4v .mp4	Various video files	These are all examples of video files and each have their advantages and disadvantages although all would require the correct CODEC to play on a video device such as a computer. WMV (Windows Media Video) is most easily played on IBM-PC computers; MOV was developed by Apple for Quicktime™.
.exe .app .dmg	Applications or programs	EXE is a Windows™ executable file, only used on IBM-PCs to install or run applications. APPs are technically bundles of files used by MacOS™ that includes a "Unix Executable File." DMG is an Apple™ disk image that commonly used in MacOS™ to install an application.
.zip, .gz, .tar, .7z	Archive	Files can be compressed into one large file using these archive types. There are programs that can be used to create these files and open these files. This process can be helpful when a large number of files needs to be backed-up or transferred.
.htm .html	Hyper-text Markup Language	Common file type that includes information to be viewed in a web browser. Most of the content found and accessed on the Internet involves this type of file. When navigating to a web page, the Internet browser often times accessing this file and reading its contents. The browser can perform functions on that page or be redirected to another page.
.sce, .psd, .ai, .logic	Proprietary or exclusive file types	A simulations operations specialist will almost certainly encounter file types that have an unfamiliar extension. An operations specialist should refer to the manufacturers or developers website for information on these types of files. Many times these files will not be readable by any program other than the program to which they are associated.

APPENDIX 5

RESOURCES FOR MOULAGE, PROPS, AND SOUNDS

EMILY SHAW

Mimic Technologies, Simugreat, SAGES, Baltimore, MD, USA

- Merica, B. J. (2011). *Medical moulage: How to make your simulations come alive*. Philadelphia, PA: F.A. Davis.
- Laerdal presentation on moulage by Sheri Howard RN, MSN, University of Memphis, Loewenberg School of Nursing:

  http://www.laerdal.com/usa/sun/presentations/14/san_diego/howard.pdf
- Moulage section of healthysimulation.com:

  http://healthysimulation.com/moulage/
- Ben Nye has bruise wheels and kits for moulage:

  http://bennye.com/
- Virginia Department of Health resources:

  http://www.moulage.net/

  http://www.fxwarehouseinc.com/

  http://www.drmass.com/casulty-simulation.html

  https://www.paintandpowderstore.com/products.php?cat=243
- Silicone mold making suppliers:

  http://www.smooth-on.com/Silicone-Rubber-an/c2_1115_1129/index.html and

  https://www.artmolds.com/molding-materials.html

Healthcare Simulation: A Guide for Operations Specialists, First Edition.
Edited by Laura T. Gantt and H. Michael Young.
© 2016 John Wiley & Sons, Inc. Published 2016 by John Wiley & Sons, Inc.

- Reference site by SSH member Kam McCowan, created for anyone in clinical simulation to use:

  http://www.behindthesimcurtain.com/moulage

  http://www.behindthesimcurtain.com/props

- Methods for recreating the insides of ambulances:

  http://www.simbulance.com/product-category/ambulance-simulators

- Posters for simulating hospital walls:

  http://simulaids.com/education/SimSpaceTrainingSupport.htm

- Headwalls:

  http://www.pocketnurse.com/Departments/Headwall

  http://www.pocketnurse.com/Departments/Simulated/

  http://www.alereusa.com/HEADWALLS.html

  http://diamedicalusa.com/nursing-school-supplies-headwall-units.php

  http://www.ghc.edu/newsarchives/srg_cd/Specifications_PDFs/11%20 70%2000_Nurse%20training%20headwall.pdf

- Pre-recorded sounds:

  https://docs.google.com/a/mimicsimulation.com/file/d/ 0B1ehFij5LyiSM2FlTXdvNlRJTms/edit

  http://www.freesound.org

  http://environment-other.ambient-mixer.com/hospital

- Recipes for making body fluids:

  http://www.laerdal.com/usa/sun/ppt/recipebook.pdf

INDEX